HERBAL
HEALING
YOUR GUIDE TO HEALING PLANTS

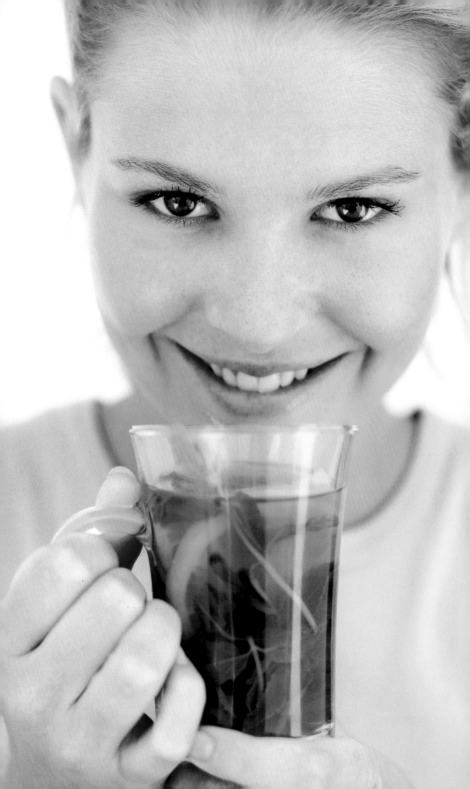

HERBAL
HEALING
YOUR GUIDE TO HEALING PLANTS

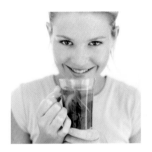

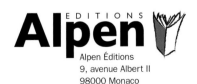

EDITIONS
Alpen
Alpen Éditions
9, avenue Albert II
98000 Monaco

Exclusive copyrights:
© Alpen Éditions
9, avenue Albert II
MC - 98000 MONACO
Tel: 00377 97 77 62 10
Fax: 00377 97 77 62 11
Web: www.alpen.mc

Managing Publisher: Christophe Didierlaurent
Editorial: Fabienne Desmarets and Sandra Del Barba
Designer: Stéphane Falaschi

Copyrights:
Catherine Martin, BSIP, Fotolia, PhotoAlto

ISBN13: 978-2-35934-074-7

Printed in Italy

Naturally Better

After centuries of evolution, knowledge and technical progress, man has re-discovered nature. This «re-discovery» is called phytotherapy and with it we have found again the roots of our natural health.

Today, its proven efficacy and incontestable benefits for our health has let phytotherapy enter our lives. We have produced this guide to help you understand better the preventive and curative principles of medicinal plants.

In the first part of this book you will find various problems that may be treated with one or a combination of medicinal plants. In the second part you will find more information on the principal plants used in phytotherapy and their traditional properties.

TABLE OF CONTENTS

PHYTOTHERAPY, NATURAL MEDICINE

The roots of medicine

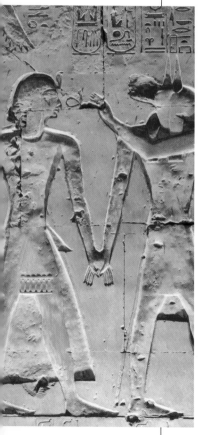

The first ever text written about medicinal plants was written on tablets of clay. There is a string of engraved tablets written by the Sumerians in about 3,000 BC. This is when the official story of phytotherapy began, although we know men used plants in the early times to feed themselves and as a remedy for their ailments.

Since then, from ancient Egyptian scientists to mystic druids, from Middle Age Chinese doctors to the great scientists of the 18th century, man has never stopped extending his knowledge of plants, their secrets and healing virtues. Old remedies and ancestral empiricism have become the science of the 21st century.

Today, scientific progress is such that new horizons on phytotherapy are forever opening: new scientific methods to understand the action of active principles of plants, to discover new properties and more practical forms for utilisation, to fit in with the needs of today's lifestyle.

A medicine for health

Phytotherapy can be differentiated from orthodox pharmaceutical remedies. There is a place for each. It is true that classic pharmaceutical remedies were favoured for nearly a century, and provided us with excellent results. Nevertheless, it is now recognized that side-effects can be experienced and people have become aware of the possible dangers of potent chemical medicines.

That is why we can now talk about two different types of medicines. Classical medicines have a strong and powerful action against illnesses and are medicines of health and well being; phytotherapy provides a gentle and often preventive action to deal with minor and chronic ailments such as arthrosis or insomnia.

With its gentle but profound action, phytotherapy is not agressive to the body but helps by stimulating the natural defences so that the benefits are more effective long-term and it has an excellent tolerance.

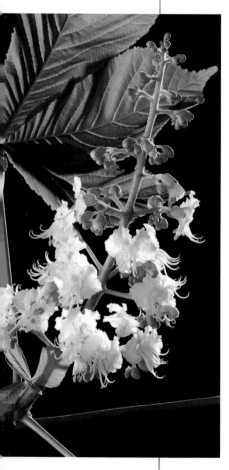

Why does phytotherapy blossom?

The world recognizes phytotherapy and it cannot be put down to fashion alone.

Of course, our era has been deeply marked by the search for a healthier lifestyle and a return to nature, but the success of phytotherapy is more readily explained by the technical and scientific progress already achieved in this area.

The progress in agronomy, chemistry and pharmacology has created safer and more efficient therapeutic formulas. With its gentle but profound action, phytotherapy is the ideal solution for modern ailments such as stress, sleep loss or overweight.

A fundamental innovation: 100% gelatin-free capsules

The development of the 100% Gelatin-Free capsule is a veritable revolution in the health sector. It is the result of lengthy research by scientific and technical teams.

Gelatin-Free capsules are made of a cellulose derivative, a natural substance which encloses and protects the cells of plants, trees, fruit and vegetables, and they provide patients with the quality, safety and harmlessness that they have a right to expect from modern medicine. This is a return to Nature's purity.

There is no visible difference between a standard capsule and a 100% Gelatin-Free capsule. This is why you should insist on the 100% Gelatin-Free capsule label. It guarantees that you are getting a reliable, quality product.

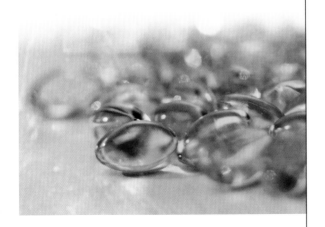

PHYTOTHERAPY: HOW TO USE IT

The best from the earth

The efficacy of phytomedicines is due to the choice of the plants used and selected. With the help of phytochemists, who have studied and researched the plants and who have identified all the precious substances within, they can be easily identified as to which one belongs to the same group and can determine with total precision as to when is the best time to harvest.

They can also determine the most favorable conditions for cultivation, the best growing areas, the best soil and of course climate. By doing this we can make sure that no fertilizers are used. It is vital that the best part of the plant, i.e. that part of the plant which has the most active ingredients, can be chosen. All plants have various active parts and some only one. The root from Harpagophytum is more active for the treatment of rheumatism and for example, in the case of Bilberry, the fruit is used against diarrhoea and the leaves to relieve haemorrhoids, so the selection of plants is based on rigorous scientific studies. «Old wives remedies» are slowly being replaced by modern sciences such as phytotherapy.

How to use plants?

Traditionally plants were infused and although this is not without a certain charm, it was quite obvious we needed a more modern form which guarantees constant efficacy, easy use and perfect hygiene. Today, this form exists in a more practical and totally controlled manner, namely the cryoground whole plant powder. A whole plant powder in a capsule easy to swallow and without flavour.

Cryogrinding - explained

This is a process using a grinder chilled with liquid nitrogen at -196°C, pulverizing the active dry part of the plant. Why are the plants frozen? Because studies have proven that the normal grinding process causes high temperatures which partly destroy the thermosensitive constituents such as vitamins, enzymes, volatile substances and numerous active principles. This does not happen with cryogrinding.

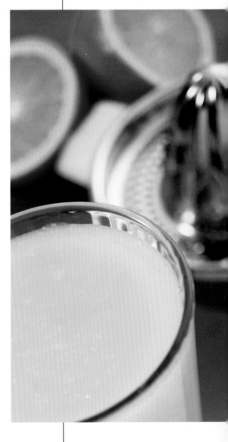

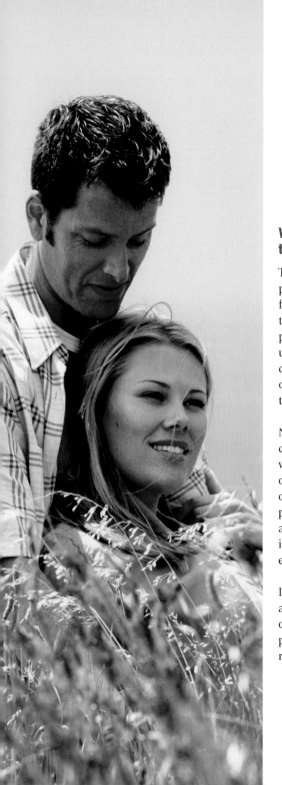

Whole plant powder: total efficacy

The advantage of the complete powder compared with other forms is that it respects all of the active constituents of the plant and brings them totally unaltered to the body. Through cryogenic grinding, the integrity of constituents is all kept within the plant powder.

None of these constituents are destroyed or suppressed. You will find in a capsule the extraordinary richness and fullness of the whole plant: its active principles, of course, but also all the constituents which act in synergy to provide a total efficacy.

In the case of plants whose activity is due to an essential oil, only the cryoground total powder is able to release entirely its beneficial effects.

Phytotherapy, your medicine

Thanks to its gentle action and better tolerance, modern phytotherapy is your daily ally. From now on, thanks to this guide, you can use all these active principles, choosing the combination of plants best adapted to your ailment.

Phytotherapy, the medicine for all the family

Children, too, can experience phytotherapy's benefits. One needs to simply adjust the dose to one capsule per 20 kg bodyweight per day. It is recommended to ask the advice of your doctor or pharmacist.

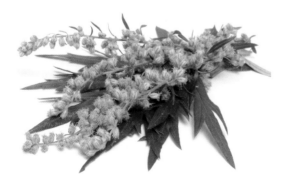

HEALTHY PLANTS FOR HEALTH PROBLEMS

	PROBLEMS	PLANTS USED	DIRECTIONS FOR USE	TREATMENT
CHOLESTEROL	CARDIOVASCULAR DISEASES (PREVENTION) CHOLESTEROL	ORGANIC FLAX OIL	1 capsule morning, noon and evening	1 month, may be repeated
		ALFALFA	1 capsule morning, noon and evening	3 months, may be repeated
	CHOLESTEROL AND HYPERTENSION	OLIVE + FISH OIL	1 capsule of each morning, noon and evening	3 months, may be repeated
		SOYA SAPONINS	1 capsule morning and evening	until troubles disappear
	DIABETES (non insulin-dependant)	BILBERRY + GREAT BURDOCK	2 capsules of each morning, noon and evening	3 months, may be repeated
		SOYA SAPONINS	1 capsule morning and evening	until troubles disappear
	TRIGLYCERIDES (excess)	ISPAGHULA	1 capsule morning, noon and evening	2 months, may be repeated
	HEART PROBLEMS	HAWTHORN	1 capsule morning, noon and evening	1 month, may be repeated
CIRCULATION	AGEING (against)	GINKGO	1 capsule morning, noon and evening	3 months, may be repeated
	ATHEROSCLEROSIS	GINKGO + BAMBOO GUM	1 capsule of each morning, noon and evening	2 months, may be repeated
	BLOOD FLUIDITY	WITCH HAZEL + GINKGO	1 capsule of each morning, noon and evening	1 month, may be repeated
	CAPILLARY FRAGILITY (frequent bruising)	BILBERRY	1 capsule morning, noon and evening	1 month, may be repeated
	CEREBRAL CIRCULATION	GINKGO	1 capsule morning, noon and evening	3 months, may be repeated
	HAEMORRHOIDS	WITCH HAZEL	2 capsules morning and evening	1 month, renewable
	MEMORY	SIBERIAN GINSENG + GINKGO	1 capsule of each morning, noon and evening	2 months, renewable
	PHLEBITIS	WITCH HAZEL + PINEAPPLE	1 capsule of each morning and evening	Until symptoms disappear
	SENESCENCE	GINKGO + BAMBOO GUM	1 capsule of each morning and evening	2 months, may be repeated
	SWOLLEN LEGS	BILBERRY + PINEAPPLE	1 capsule of each morning, noon and evening	1 month, may be repeated
	TIRED LEGS	WITCH HAZEL	2 capsules morning and evening	1 month, renewable
	VARICOSE VEINS	BILBERRY + WITCH HAZEL	1 capsule of each morning, noon and evening	1 month, may be repeated

DERMATOLOGY - SKIN

PROBLEMS	PLANTS USED	DIRECTIONS FOR USE	TREATMENT
ACNE	GREAT BURDOCK	2 capsules twice a day	1 to 3 months
ALLERGIC ECZEMA	PLANTAIN + GREAT BURDOCK	1 capsule of each morning and evening	1 month, renewable
BRITTLE NAILS AND HAIR	BAMBOO GUM + ALFALFA	1 capsule of each morning, noon and evening	3 months, may be repeated
ECZEMA	GREAT BURDOCK + starflower oil	1 capsule of each morning and evening	1 month, renewable
EXCESSIVE PERSPIRATION	SAGE	2 capsules morning and evening	1 month, renewable
dry SKIN	evening primrose oil + starflower oil	1 capsule of each morning and noon	2 months, may be repeated
HAIR LOSS	STINGING NETTLE + BAMBOO GUM	1 capsule of each morning, noon and evening	3 months, may be repeated
PSORIASIS	CALIFORNIAN POPPY + BAMBOO GUM	1 capsule of each morning, noon and evening	3 months, may be repeated
ROSACEA (skin blotches)	WITCH HAZEL + BILBERRY	1 capsule of each morning, noon and evening	1 month, may be repeated
SKIN BEAUTY	starflower oil	1 of starflower oil a day	may be repeated
SKIN ageing (prevention)	starflower oil + ginkgo	1 capsule of each morning and noon	2 months, may be repeated
Stretch marks	starflower oil	1 capsule morning and noon	1 month, renewable
URTICARIA	CALIFORNIAN POPPY + PLANTAIN	1 capsule of each noon and evening	3 weeks, may be repeated
VISUAL ACUITY	BILBERRY	1 capsule morning, noon and evening	3 months, may be repeated
wrinkles	starflower oil + ginkgo	2 capsules of each morning and noon	2 months, may be repeated

DIGESTION

PROBLEMS	PLANTS USED	DIRECTIONS FOR USE	TREATMENT
AEROPHAGY	CHARCOAL	1 capsule morning, noon and evening	Until troubles disappear
BAD BREATH	CHARCOAL	1 capsule morning, noon and evening	15 days, repeatable
CHRONIC CONSTIPATION	ISPAGHULA	3 capsules 1 hour before lunch and dinner	Maintain treatment over several months
DIARRHOEA	BILBERRY + ISPAGHULA	1 capsule of each morning and evening	Until troubles disappear
DIGESTION (difficult)	PINEAPPLE + SAGE	1 capsule of each morning, noon and evening	10 days
FLATULENCE	SAGE	2 capsules before	1 to 2 weeks
FOOD POISONING	MILK THISTLE + CHARCOAL	1 capsule of each morning, noon and evening	1 month, repeatable

PROBLEMS	PLANTS USED	DIRECTIONS FOR USE	TREATMENT
FREQUENT CONSTIPATION	ISPAGHULA	3 capsules 1 hour before lunch and dinner	15 days
GALLSTONES	ARTICHOKE	1 capsule morning, noon and evening	1 month, may be repeated
HEPATITIS (OR JAUNDICE)	ARTICHOKE + MILK THISTLE	1 capsule of each morning, noon and evening	1 month may be repeated
INTESTINAL INFECTION	ECHINACEA + SAGE	1 capsule of each morning, noon and evening	Until troubles disappear
INTESTINAL SPASMS	CALIFORNIAN POPPY + ISPAGHULA	1 capsule of each morning, noon and evening	1 month, may be repeated
LACK OF APPETITE	GINGER	2 capsules noon and evening	2 months
NAUSEA	GINGER	2 capsules per day	When necessary
OCCASIONAL CONSTIPATION	ISPAGHULA	3 capsules 1 hour before lunch and dinner	1 week
TRAVEL SICKNESS GASTRITIS	GINGER	2 capsules half an hour before journey	Repeat as necessary

Section label (vertical): DIGESTION

PROBLEMS	PLANTS USED	DIRECTIONS FOR USE	TREATMENT
ANXIETY	VALERIAN	2 capsules morning and evening	15 days
	HAWTHORN	1 capsule morning and evening	1 month, may be repeated
DEPRESSION	ST JOHN'S WORT	1 capsule at breakfast and lunch	Until troubles disappear
	RHODIOLA	1 capsule morning and noon	1 to 4 months
EMOTION	VALERIAN + PASSIFLORA	1 capsule of each morning, noon and evening	15 days, may be repeated
INSOMNIA	CALIFORNIAN POPPY + PASSIFLORA	1 capsule of each before dinner and on going to bed	1 month, may be repeated
	HAWTHORN	1 capsule morning and evening	1 month, may be repeated
NERVOUSNESS	PASSIFLORA	1 capsule morning, noon and evening	1 month, may be repeated
	HAWTHORN	1 capsule morning, noon and evening	1 month, may be repeated
NEURALGIA	CALIFORNIAN POPPY	2 capsules morning and evening	1 to 2 weeks
NIGHTMARES	CALIFORNIAN POPPY	2 capsules before dinner and on going to bed	Until troubles disappear
OVERWORK	SIBERIAN GINSENG + PASSIFLORA	2 capsules of each morning and noon	1 month, may be repeated
STRESS	VALERIAN	2 capsules morning and evening	1 month, may be repeated

Section label (vertical): INSOMNIA - NERVOUSNESS

P A I N S

PROBLEMS	PLANTS USED	DIRECTIONS FOR USE	TREATMENT
ARTHROSIS	DEVIL'S CLAW + BAMBOO GUM	1 capsule of each morning, noon and evening	3 months, may be repeated
BACK PAINS	DEVIL'S CLAW	2 capsules morning and evening	15 days
CARTILAGE (wear or disappearance)	STINGING NETTLE + BAMBOO GUM	1 capsule of each morning, noon and evening	2 months, renewable
FRACTURES (consolidation of)	BAMBOO	1 capsule morning, noon and evening	1 month, repeatable
GOUT	STINGING NETTLE + DEVIL'S CLAW	1 capsule of each morning, noon and evening	2 months, may be repeated
HEADACHES	CALIFORNIAN POPPY + FEVERFEW	1 capsule of each morning, noon and evening	Until relief is obtained
JOINT PAINS	DEVIL'S CLAW	3 capsules morning, noon and evening	15 days, may be repeated
MIGRAINE	FEVERFEW	2 capsules in the morning	1 month
MIGRAINE (prevention)	FEVERFEW	1 capsule in the morning	2 months
OSTEOPOROSIS	ALFALFA + BAMBOO GUM	1 capsule of each morning, noon and evening	3 months, may be repeated
RHEUMATISM	DEVIL'S CLAW + BAMBOO GUM	1 capsule of each morning, noon and evening	3 months, may be repeated
SCIATICA	DEVIL'S CLAW	1 capsule after breakfast, lunch and dinner	2 weeks
SPRAINS	DEVIL'S CLAW + PINEAPPLE	1 capsule of each morning, noon and evening	Until relief is obtained
TENDINITIS	DEVIL'S CLAW	1 capsule morning, noon and evening	1 month, repeatable

O T H E R

SMOKING (breaking the habit)	VALERIAN	2 capsules morning, and evening	1 month, may be repeated
VIRAL DISORDERS	ECHINACEA	2 capsules morning, noon and evening	Until relief is obtained

	PROBLEMS	PLANTS USED	DIRECTIONS FOR USE	TREATMENT
R E S P I R A T O R Y	ALLERGIES	PLANTAIN	1 capsule 3 times per day	1 month, may be repeated
	ASTHMA	PLANTAIN	2 capsules twice a day	1 month may be repeated
	CHRONIC BRONCHITIS	ECHINACEA + PLANTAIN	2 capsules of each morning and evening	1 month, may be repeated
	COLDS	ECHINACEA + GUARANA	2 capsules of each morning and evening	10 days
	HAY FEVER	PLANTAIN	1 capsule morning, noon and evening	As long as necessary
		EYEBRIGHT COMMON PLANTAIN BITTER ORANGE	1 capsule every hour (up to 8 capsules/day) for 3 days, then, 1 capsule morning and evening	As long as necessary
	INFLUENZA	ECHINACEA + SIBERIAN GINSENG	2 capsules of each morning and evening	2 to 3 weeks

	PROBLEMS	PLANTS USED	DIRECTIONS FOR USE	TREATMENT
S L I M M I N G	APPETITE SUPPRESSANT	ISPAGHULA + SEAWEED	2 capsules of ispaghula and 1 capsule of seaweed half an hour before every meal	As much as necessary
	CELLULITE	GREEN TEA + PINEAPPLE	1 capsule of each morning, noon and evening	2 months, may be repeated
	FLUID RETENTION	STINGING NETTLE + GREEN TEA	1 capsule of each morning, noon and evening	2 months, may be repeated
		SOYA SAPONINS	1 capsule morning and evening	until troubles disappear
	OBESITY (WITH A LARGE APPETITE)	GUARANA + GREEN TEA + ISPAGHULA	1 capsule of each morning and noon	10 weeks, may be repeated
		SOYA SAPONINS	1 capsule morning and evening	until troubles disappear
	OVERWEIGHT (SLIGHT)	GREEN TEA ISPAGHULA	1 capsule of each morning, noon and evening	10 weeks, may be repeated
	WEIGHT CONTROL	GUARANA + SEAWEED	1 capsule of each morning, noon and evening	3 weeks, may be repeated
		RHODIOLA	1 capsule morning and noon	1 to 4 months
		NOPAL CACTUS	1 capsule morning, noon and evening and 2 capsules after heavy meals	1 month, may be repeated

HEALTHY PLANTS FOR HEALTH PROBLEMS

PROBLEMS	PLANTS USED	DIRECTIONS FOR USE	TREATMENT
APHRODISIAC	DAMIANA + GINGER	2 capsules of each morning and evening	1 month, may be repeated
SPORT	SIBERIAN GINSENG GUARANA RHODIOLA	1 capsule of each morning, noon and evening 1 capsule morning and noon	1 month, may be repeated 1 to 4 months
EXHAUSTION	SIBERIAN GINSENG + SEAWEED	2 capsules of each morning and noon	1 month, may be repeated
SEXUAL TIREDNESS	SIBERIAN GINSENG + DAMIANA + GINGER	1 capsule of each morning and noon	1 month, may be repeated
INTELLECTUAL FATIGUE	SIBERIAN GINSENG + GINKGO RHODIOLA	1 capsule of each morning, noon and evening 1 capsule morning and noon	1 month, may be repeated 1 to 4 months
PHYSICAL FATIGUE	GUARANA + SEAWEED SOYA SAPONINS	1 capsule of each morning, noon and evening 1 capsule morning and noon	1 month, may be repeated until troubles disappear
NERVOUS TIREDNESS	PASSIFLORA + GUARANA	1 capsule of each morning, noon and evening	1 month, may be repeated

PROBLEMS	PLANTS USED	DIRECTIONS FOR USE	TREATMENT
DEPURATIVE	GREAT BURDOCK STINGING NETTLE	1 capsule of each morning, noon and evening	Until an improvment is obtained
	CHERRY STALK	2 capsules morning and midday	3 weeks, may be repeated
DIURETIC	STINGING NETTLE + GREEN TEA	1 capsule of each morning, noon and evening	Until an improvment is obtained
	CHERRY STALK	2 capsules morning and midday	3 weeks, may be repeated
ENURESIS (Bed wetting)	CALIFORNIAN POPPY + SIBERIAN GINSENG	1 capsule of each morning and evening	Until an improvment is obtained
PROSTATE (hypertrophy)	PUMPKIN SEED/ SAW PALMETTO	2 capsules a day	2 months, may be repeated
	SOYA ISOFLAVONES PLANT STEROLS/ZINC	1 capsule morning and evening	1 month, may be repeated
CYSTITIS	CRANBERRY + Vitamin C	2 capsules morning and evening during 10 days, then 1 capsule morning and evening	1 month, may be repeated

PROBLEMS	PLANTS USED	DIRECTIONS FOR USE	TREATMENT
HOT FLUSHES	SAGE SOYA ISOFLAVONES	2 capsules twice a day 2 capsules a day	Until troubles disappear
	BLACK COHOSH	2 capsules in the evening	Until troubles disappear
IRREGULAR MENSTRUATION	EVENING PRIMROSE OIL + SAGE	1 capsule of each morning and evening	During the 2nd half of the cycle
MENOPAUSE TROUBLES	SAGE + ALFALFA	1 capsule of each morning, noon and evening	2 months, may be repeated
	BLACK COHOSH	2 capsules in the evening	Until troubles disappear
PAINFUL MENSTRUATION	EVENING PRIMROSE OIL + SAGE	1 capsule of each morning and evening	During the 2nd half of the cycle
PREMENSTRUAL SYNDROME	EVENING PRIMROSE OIL + SAGE	1 capsule of each morning and evening	During the 2nd half of the cycle
TENDERNESS OF THE BREASTS	EVENING PRIMROSE OIL	1 capsule morning and evening	During the 2nd half of the cycle

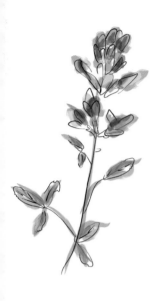

PLANTS
THE ESSENTIAL MINERALISATION

ALFALFA
Medicago sativa

Part used: leaf sap

This common plant found in the temperate areas of Europe has nutritive and remineralising properties.

In fact it contains a very high content of proteins, (which can be up to 55%), amino acids (which make up proteins), vitamins, trace elements, such as calcium, iron, phosphorus, zinc, copper, selenium and silica. With its content of iron, it is particularly recommended for anaemia and asthenia.

All its nutrients are of benefit to the growth and the strengthening of nails and hair.

The latest studies show that a regular intake has a moderate hypocholesterolemic and atherosclerosis preventive action.

The presence of a vegetal oestrogen (coumestrol) with its hormonal action coupled with the remineralising properties of silica and calcium, helps reduce the troubles linked to the menopause and osteoporosis.

Recommended for:
- Brittle nails and hair
- Asthenia, anaemia
- Osteoporosis and menopause
- Prevention of cardiovascular diseases.

DOSAGE
435mg per capsule of total plant cryoground powder

PHYTO PRESCRIPTION
Take 1 capsule morning, noon and evening during meals with a large glass of water.

Contraindications/ Side-effects:
None known.

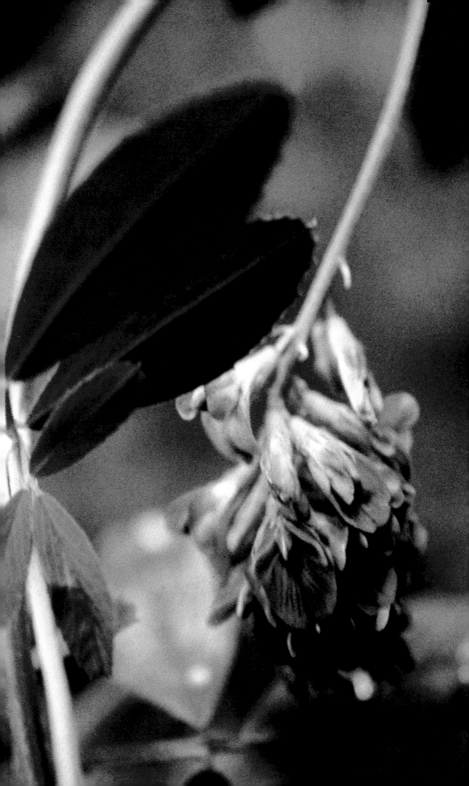

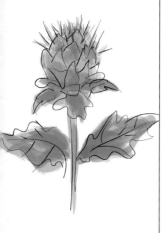

POOR DIGESTION
HEPATOBILIARY DISORDERS
CONSTIPATION DUE TO HEPATIC
INSUFFICIENCY

ARTICHOKE
Cynara scolymus

Part used: leaf

Originating in North Africa and cultivated in France, artichoke is a majestic plant of which the flower bud is eaten, whereas phytotherapy uses the leaves to treat liver and gall bladder diseases. The major component in the leaf is cynarin, which is amphocholeretic, i.e. it stimulates both formation and elimination of bile. Artichoke leaf is thus used to treat liver and gall bladder disorders. It is a liver protector and liver cell regenerator used in icterus (jaundice) and its sequelae, also in cirrhotics to stimulate liver renewal. Artichoke being a choleretic, it makes it possible to combat constipation related to hepatic insufficiency. In addition to cynarin, artichoke leaf contains a number of substances which potentiate its beneficial action on the liver, thus the therapeutic utility of employing a cryoground whole powder of this plant to obtain the total benefits of all its constituents. It is also hypocholesterolemic and slightly hypotensive.

Recommended for:
- Poor digestion
- Hepatobiliary disorders
- Constipation due to hepatic insufficiency

DOSAGE
200mg per capsule of total plant cryoground powder

PHYTO PRESCRIPTION
1 capsule morning, noon and evening,
to be taken before meals.
Contraindications/ Side-effects:
None known.

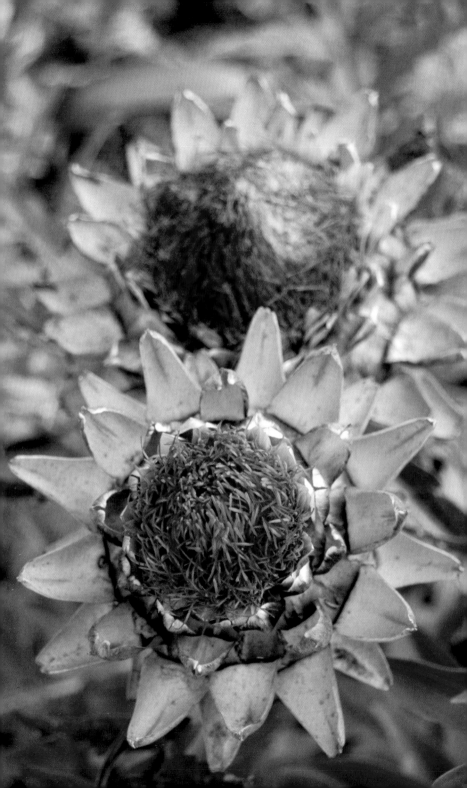

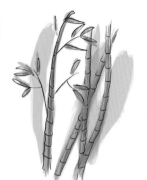

BAMBOO GUM
Bambousa arundinacea

Part used: siliceous concretion of bamboo stem

Bamboo is an exotic reed which grows very quickly and sometimes up to over twenty centimetres a day and can measure up to ten metres. It is often used as building material in Asia. In natural medicine, the siliceous secretion is harvested on the knots of the stems which are called bamboosil or Tabashir in India and China.

Being very rich in silica, bamboo gum has a beneficial action on the joints, it stimulates the synthesis of collagen in the bones and connective tissues thus facilitating the reconstitution of the cartilage which can be destroyed during articular illnesses. With its remineralising properties, it can also help prevent bone loss brought on by the menopause.

Recommended for:
- Remineralising
- Backache
- Osteoporosis

DOSAGE
320mg per capsule of total plant cryoground powder

PHYTO PRESCRIPTION
Take 1 capsule morning, noon and evening during meals with a large glass of water

Contraindications/ Side-effects:
None known.

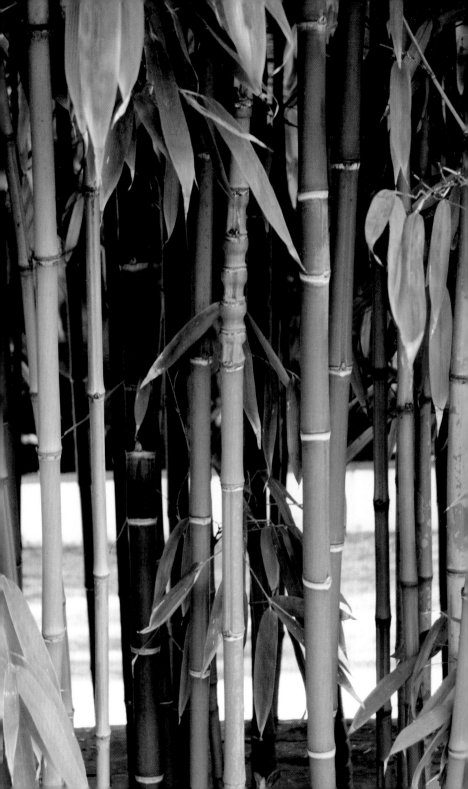

A TONIC FOR YOUR VEINS

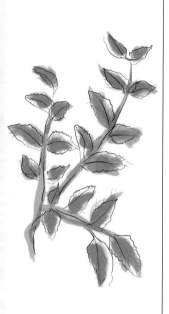

BILBERRY LEAVES

Vaccinium myrtillus

Part used: the leaf

Bilberry leaves are sharp and oval-shaped and contain flavonic polyphenols. These flavonoids provide the leaves with vitamin P properties: they increase the resistance of the capillaries, regulate their permeability and also act as an anti-inflammatory.

The condensed tannins they contain are astringent and angio-protectors. With their various properties, Bilberry leaves are recommended for microcirculation problems. It is interesting to note the hypoglycaemic action for mild and non-insulin dependent diabetes. They could also be used for diabetes linked to ageing.

Recommended for:
- Capillary fragility
- Rosacea (skin blotches)
- Non-insulin dependent diabetes
- Diabetes linked to ageing

DOSAGE
320mg per capsule of total plant cryoground powder

PHYTO PRESCRIPTION
Take 1 capsule morning, noon and evening during meals with a large glass of water. The intake can be increased to 5 capsules per day

Contraindications/ Side-effects:
None known.

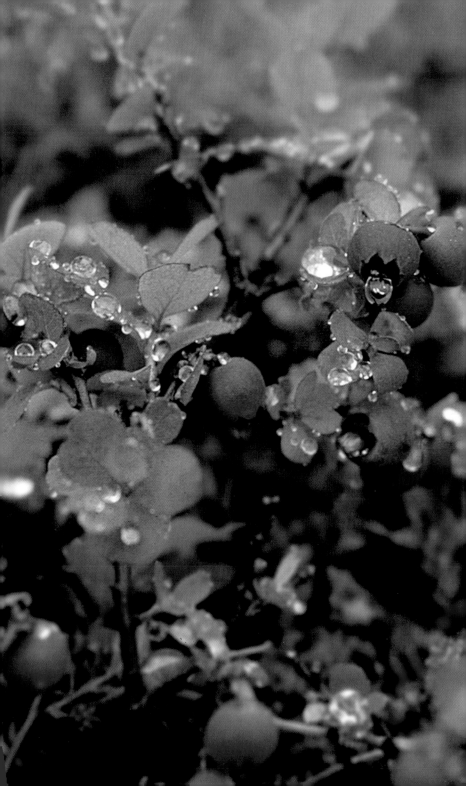

BLACK COHOSH
Cimicifuga racemosa

Part used: Roots

Black cohosh is a perennial wildflower native to Eastern North America. Native Americans and early colonists used Black Cohosh root to treat conditions including general malaise, malaria, rheumatism, sore throat, menstrual irregularities.

Black Cohosh has been used in Europe for more than 40 years to treat symptoms associated with menopause, by regulating the pituitary's secretion of lutenising hormone, the primary cause of hot flushes. The herb appears to display an oestrogen-like effect, binding to oestrogen receptors in the body. Currently, Black Cohosh root is approved by the German Government to treat premenstrual discomfort, painful menstruation, and menopausal symptoms.

Recommended for:
- Menopausal symptoms: hot flushes, heart palpitations, nervousness and irritability, sleep disturbances and depression.
- Premenstrual discomfort
- Dysmenorrhea

DOSAGE
360mg of powdered Black Cohosh root

PHYTO PRESCRIPTION
1 capsule in the evening with a large glass of water.

Contraindications/ Side-effects:
Pregnant and/or lactating patients should not use Black Cohosh. It is not recommended during pregnancy because it may promote menstrual flow or stimulate the uterus. Black Cohosh is not recommended during breast-feeding. Black Cohosh may interfere with hormonal medications, such as contraceptive pills. Avoid Black Cohosh if you are receiving medication for hypertension; it may intensify the drug's effect of lowering blood pressure.

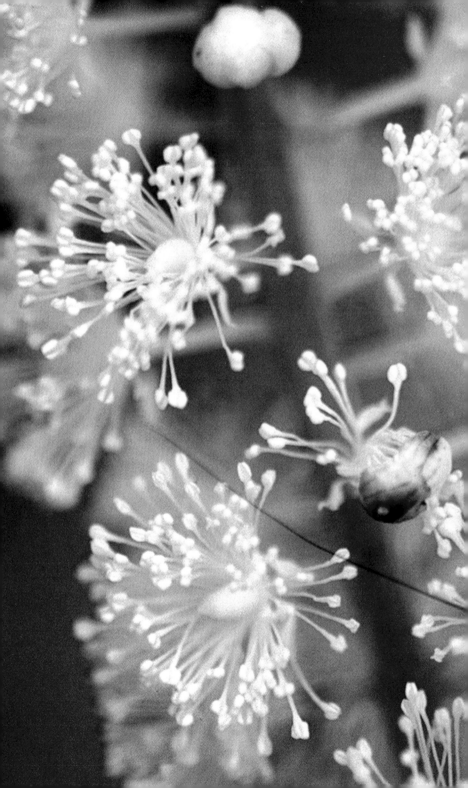

CALIFORNIAN POPPY
Eschscholtzia californica

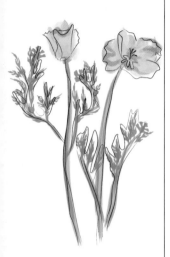

Part used: the aerial flowered part

Eschscholtzia comes from California where it covers large areas near Sequoia forests, creating a pretty yellow horizon. Californian poppy contains alkaloids and in particular one called californidine. This plant is a natural hypnotic: it prepares for peaceful sleep, reduces sleeping problems, particularly nightmares, waking during the night and difficulties in falling asleep. It is also an anxiolytic and a sedative: it helps anxious people of all ages recover and have a calm life without stress. As it has no side-effects and is nonaddictive, Californian poppy is the alternative choice to experience restful nights. This plant is also an antispasmodic: it gives good results for the treatment of colitis, acting on intestinal spasms and pains. It can also be used with great success with Ispaghula to relieve intestinal tract disorders.

Recommended for:
- Sleeping problems for both adults and children
- Anxiety, nightmares, depression
- Intestinal spasms of the colon

DOSAGE
300mg per capsule of total plant cryoground powder

PHYTO PRESCRIPTION
Take 2 capsules in the evening during meals and 2 capsules before going to bed. Children (6 to 9 years): 1 capsule before going to bed with a large glass of water Children (10-14 years): 1 capsule in the evening during meals and 1 capsule before going to bed.

Contraindications/ Side-effects:
None known.

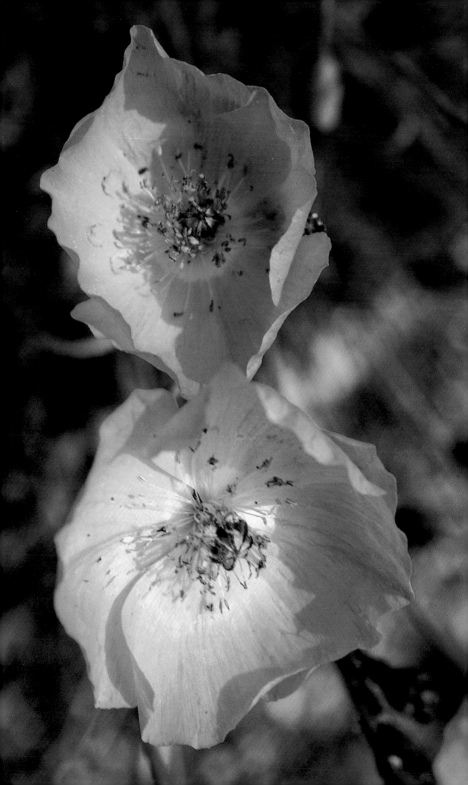

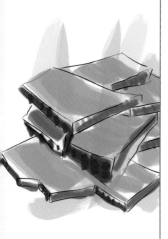

VEGETABLE CHARCOAL

Charcoal is obtained by charring coconut shells. The process makes it possible to create a whole network of pores which considerably increase the charcoal's specific adsorption surface area. It is thus the most powerful adsorbent of natural origin currently known. Charcoal passes through the digestive tract, where it is perfectly tolerated. It has the ability to adsorb, i.e. to fix on to its surface, various substances such as bacteria, toxins and gases.

It is beneficial for the treatment of functional disorders of the digestive system such as abdominal pains, transit disorders and distension. Activated charcoal efficiently controls aerophagy, eructations (belching) and intestinal gases. Charcoal thus helps to improve the figure by recovering a flat stomach. Similarly, charcoal stops bad breath, generally due to excessive intestinal fermentation.

Finally, it is useful in the treatment of diarrhoea because it adsorbs bacteria and forms an intestinal coating.

Recommended for:
- Aerophagy
- Bad breath
- Abdominal pains

DOSAGE
162mg per capsule

PHYTO PRESCRIPTION
Adults: 4 capsules per day, to be taken between meals. Children aged 6-15: 1-4 capsules per day.

Contraindications/ Side-effects:

Those currently on medication should leave at least a gap of 2 hours between this product and their medicines.

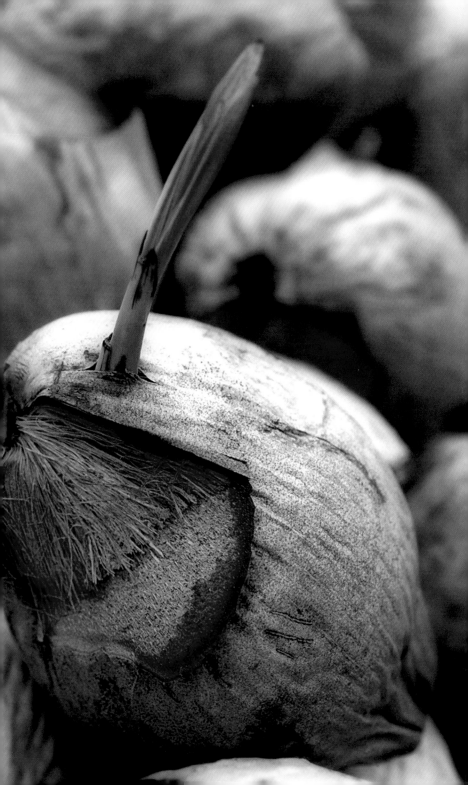

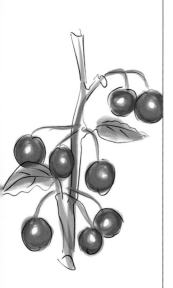

DIURETIC AND DEPURATIVE

CHERRY STALK
Prunus cerasus

Part used: the peduncle of the fruit

Known and used for centuries as a depurative and diuretic, cherry stalk is especially valued nowadays for its safe diuretic action, free from unwanted effects.

It allows cleansing of the whole body by eliminating accumulated toxins. The flavonoids and potassium salts that it contains promote renal water elimination and combat the urinary tract inflammation that occurs during urinary infections.

It is an aid in the treatment of oedema, urinary calculi (stones that may block the urinary tract), cystitis and slight hypertension because of its diuresis-stimulating effect.

Recommended for:
- Water retention
- Detoxification
- Urinary problems
- Hypertension

DOSAGE
350mg per capsule of total plant cryoground powder

PHYTO PRESCRIPTION
2 capsules morning and midday, to be taken at mealtimes.

Contraindications/ Side-effects:
None known.

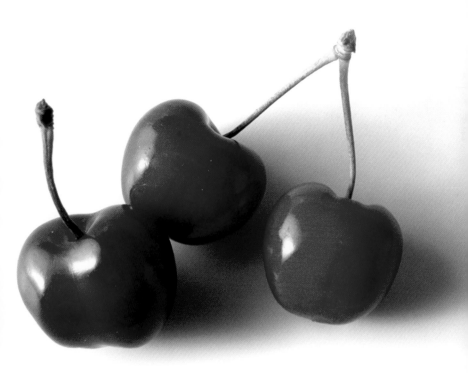

CRANBERRY + VITAMIN C

Vaccinium Macrocarpon
Malpighia Glabra

Part used: fruit

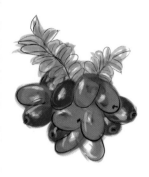

Cranberry is a bitter red berry derived from a low-lying evergreen (-Vacciniun Macrocarpon-) native to North America. Cranberry's can assist in the prevention and alleviate urinary tract infections. It is a relatively modern discovery dating from the early twentieth century. Cranberry prevents E. Coli, the most common cause of urinary tract infections and recurrent urinary tract infections, from adhering to the cells lining the wall of the bladder.

This anti-adhesive action renders the bacteria harmless in the urinary tract. The constituents in Cranberry responsible for this anti-adhesive activity have yet to be identified.

Taking natural Vitamin C contained in Acerola berries (Malpighia Glabra), at the same time, enhances the efficacy of Cranberry.

Recommended for:

• To prevent and treat urinary tract infections and cystitis

DOSAGE

450mg per capsule of total plant cryoground powder

PHYTO PRESCRIPTION

Initial intake: take 2 capsules in the morning and evening during meals with a large glass of water, for a period of 10 days.
Then, take 1 capsule in the morning and evening during meals
with a large glass of water.

Contraindications/
Side-effects:

No known side-effects have been reported when taking Cranberry concentrate. It is safe for use during pregnancy and lactation. Cranberry should not be used as a substitute for antibiotics during an acute urinary infection.

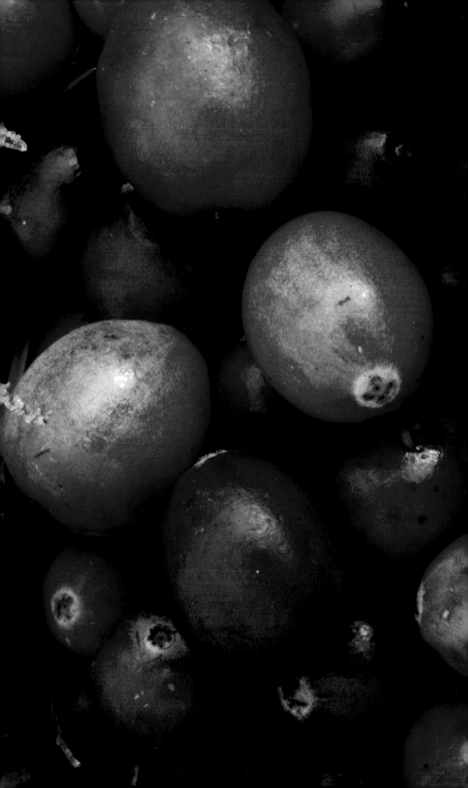

DAMIANA
Turnera aphrodisiaca

Part used: leaves and stem

Damiana is a small shrub which grows in Mexico, Texas and parts of South America. Originating from its use by Mexican Indians, Damiana has a time-honoured reputation, widely mentioned in literature, as an aphrodisiac.

It owes its properties to a greenish volatile oil, which smells like chamomile and a bitter substance called damianin. Damiana is also used in cases of overwork, mental stress and nervous debility.

Recommended for:
- Sexual disorders
- Aphrodisiac
- Depressive states
- Constipation.

DOSAGE
325mg per capsule of total plant cryoground powder

PHYTO PRESCRIPTION
Take 1 capsule morning, noon and evening during meals with a large glass of water.
Contraindications/ Side-effects:
None known.

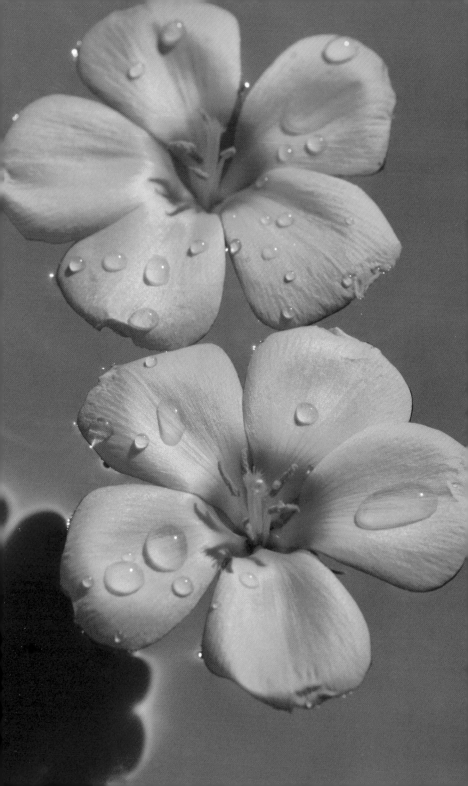

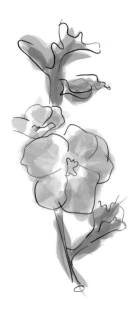

A TREATMENT FOR JOINT PAINS AND HELPS CREATE FLEXIBILITY

DEVIL'S CLAW
Harpagophytum procumbens

Part used: the secondary roots

Harpagophytum is a South African, creeping plant. It grows in Namibia and has been used for centuries by the local healers to treat pain and inflammation of the joints. Its fruit has hooked thorns which has given the plant its common name "Devil's claw". The part we use comes from secondary roots. They are rich in glucoiridoids and in particular harpagoside. They have wonderful antiinflammatory properties and are a great treatment for rheumatism and arthritis. They act on the pain and inflammation thus improving joint mobility. Devil's claw can be used to progressively replace traditional antiinflammatory treatments because it has no side-effects. Sports people often use Devil's claw with great success to help them avoid tendon and articular pain, caused by intensive sporting efforts. Devil's claw root will also favour uric acid elimination and it is therefore an efficient treatment for problems related to gout. Numerous clinical studies have confirmed these properties.

To gain full effectiveness it can be purchased in capsules for oral consumption and is also available as a gel for atopic massage.

Recommended for:
- Rheumatism
- Arthritis
- Can be a complementary treatment for rheumatoid arthritis
- Tendon and articular pain for sportsmen
- Gout

DOSAGE
435mg per capsule of total plant cryoground powder

PHYTO PRESCRIPTION
Take 1 capsule morning, noon and evening during meals with a large glass of water. Intake can be increased to 6 capsules per day.

Contraindications/ Side-effects:
None known.

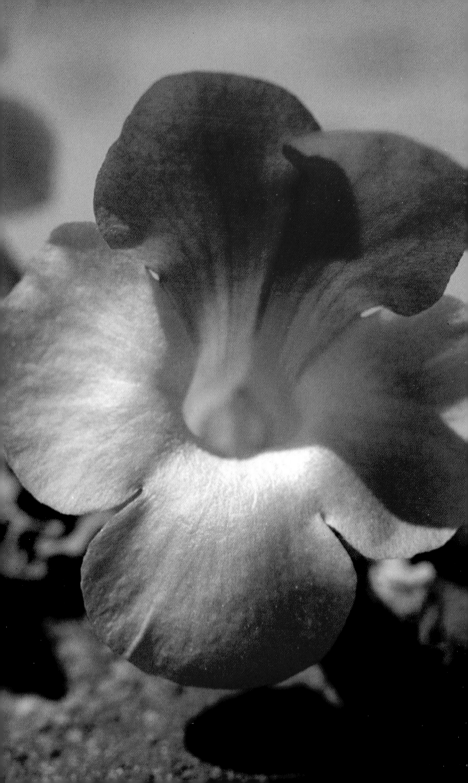

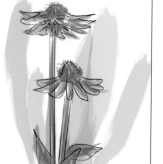

ECHINACEA
Echinacea purpurea

Part used: the root

Echinacea is a native of the U.S.A. but is also now cultivated in Britain. This plant was used by the Indians for wounds. The flowers are a rich purple in colour and are borne on a stout stem. It is the roots which are used, being of a tapered cylindrical shape with a slight spiral. One of its common names is "Sampson" root.

Echinacea root contains polysaccharides which have an immunostimulant activity. They stimulate the body's non-specific defences (1).

Echinacea is not only used for colds and influenza but also for many types of bacterial and viral infections, and skin complaints.

Recommended for:
• Colds, influenza
• Viral and bacterial disorders
• Skin complaints

DOSAGE
250mg per capsule of total plant cryoground powder

PHYTO PRESCRIPTION
Adults and elderly : 1 to 2 capsules to be taken with a glass of water before meals 3 times daily..

Contraindications/ Side-effects:
Not recommended for those with autoimmune diseases and in case of allergies to drug of the Compositae family.
Not recommended during pregnancy.

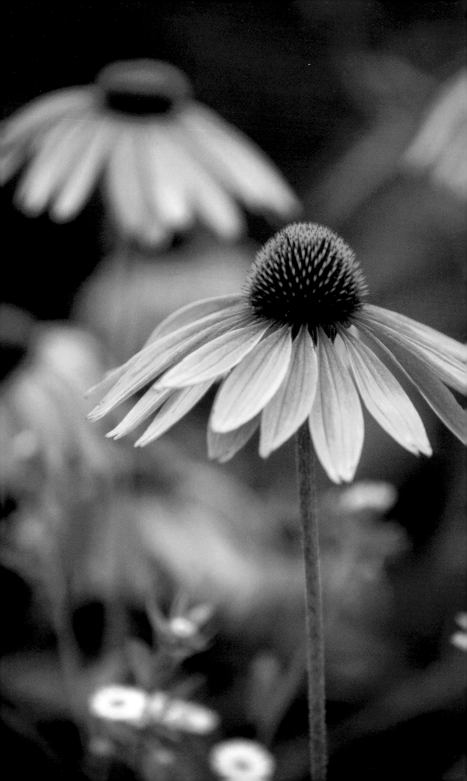

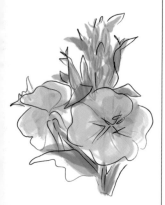

EVENING PRIMROSE OIL
Oenothera biennis

Part used: the oil extracted from the seeds

This plant carries big and beautiful yellow flowers and likes areas of moderate and mild temperature. It is often found near ponds in the Languedoc region of France. The oil extracted from the seeds by cold pressing is extremely rich in Essential Fatty Acid (E.F.A.). It contains 72% of Linoleic Acid and 10% of Gamma Linolenic Acid. These are the precursors of prostaglandins, substances that influence the menstrual cycle. Recent clinical studies have shown that E.P.O. taken during the second half of the cycle clearly reduces the pre-menstrual syndrome, working on all its different symptoms; depression, irritability, tenderness of the breasts, abdominal pains, water retention and headaches (cephalagia). These convincing results cannot be ignored by those who continuously suffer with this problem. When taken regularly, E.P.O. is also beneficial for the heart: Gamma Linolenic Acid regularises cholesterol levels and blood pressure.

Recommended for:
• Pre-menstrual syndrome: Irritability, tenderness of the breasts, water retention, abdominal pains etc...

DOSAGE
520mg per capsule of first cold pressed Evening Primrose Oil (E.P.O.)

PHYTO PRESCRIPTION
Take 1 to 3 capsules a day during meals with a large glass of water.

Contraindications/ Side-effects:
Not to be used if taking anti-coagulant drugs or if haemophilic.

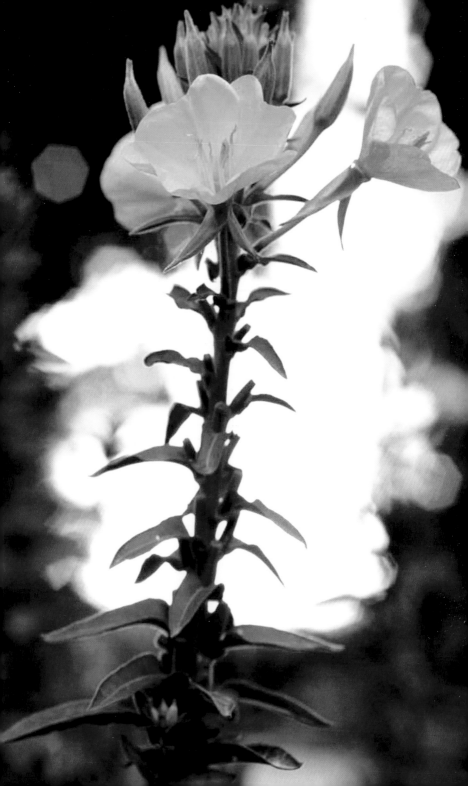

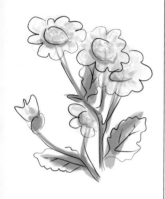

FOR THOSE WHO SUFFER FROM MIGRAINE

FEVERFEW
Tanacetum parthenium

Part used: the flowering tip

Originally from the Balkan States, this plant was introduced into Western Europe by the British. Feverfew is often referred to as the "big chamomile". Its flowering tips contain parthenolide, which contributes to its antimigraine activity.

The mechanism that often starts a migraine is now known. Different factors such as stress, emotion, food intolerance, and often menstrual conditions cause the organism to liberate a hormone called serotonin which provokes alternation of contractions and dilatations of the cerebral arteries and therefore provokes the pain. Parthenolide blocks the liberation of serotonin, efficaciously preventing the onset of migraine. A three month course permits a noticeable decrease in the frequency and intensity of migraines and relieves people suffering from this painful and often stressful ailment.

Recommended for:
• Migraines.

DOSAGE
260mg per capsule of total plant cryoground powder

PHYTO PRESCRIPTION
Take 2 capsules in the morning for 1 month, after which as a maintenance intake 1 capsule per day for 2 months.

**Contraindications/
Side-effects:**
Not recommended in case of allergies to drug of the Compositae family Not recommended during pregnancy.

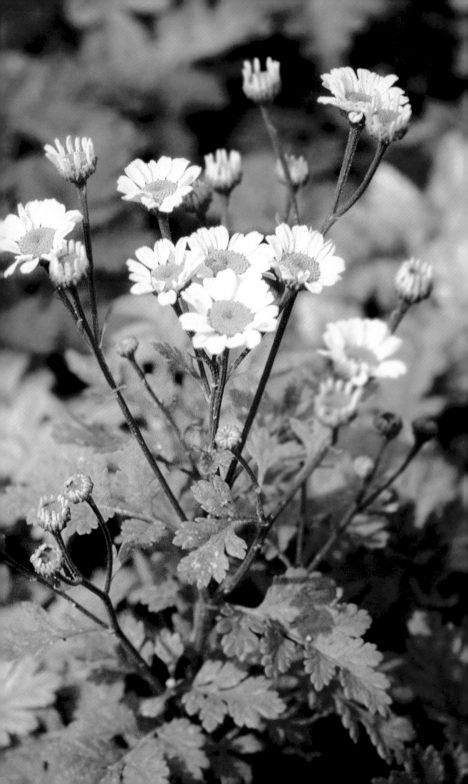

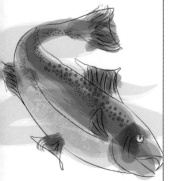

TO SUPPORT HEALTHY HEART FUNCTION AND JOINT FLEXIBILITY

FISH OIL

Fish oil provides the Omega-3 fatty acids EPA and DHA, which are as important to good health as essential vitamins and minerals. The higher the content of EFAs in the diet, the more fluid and flexible the membrane is, resulting in a more efficient exchange across the membrane. If your diet consists primarily of saturated fats and not enough Omega-3 fatty acids, your cellular membranes can stiffen and become rigid. The membrane exchanges slow down and chronic health conditions may occur.

Many clinical studies have shown the health benefits of Omega-3 fatty acids, in particular EFA and DHA. The scientific literature provides many published studies on fish oil, ranging from diabetes to heart disease. As a matter of fact, your brain actually contains 20% DHA.

The body can produce a small amount of EPA and DHA from Alpha Linolenic Acid found in the diet (flax oil, nuts, blackcurrant oil, red meat). However, many factors can impair the production of EFA and DHA, such as consumption of sugar, alcohol, saturated fats and trans fatty acids (margarine, processed food), ageing and stress, to name only a few.

Recommended for:
- Healthy heart function
- Joint flexibility

PHYTO PRESCRIPTION
1 capsule during the day, can be increased to 2 capsules per day.
Contraindications/ Side-effects:
None known.

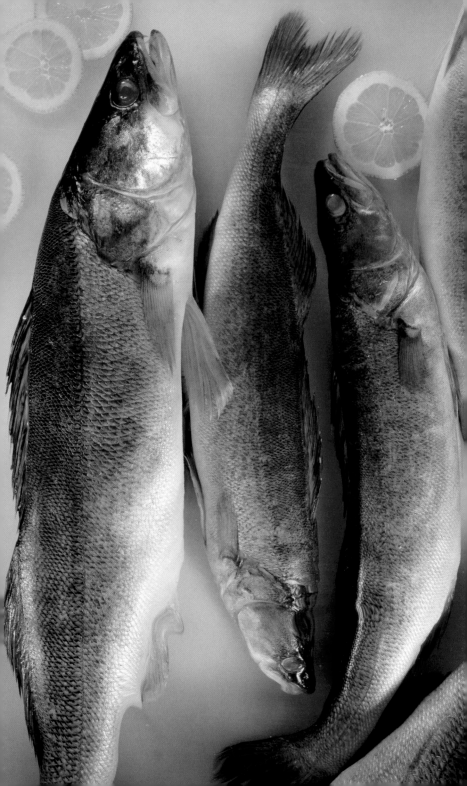

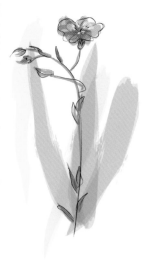

FLAX OIL
Linum usitatissimum

Part used: the oil extract from the seeds

Intestinal transit and supply of EFAs: Everyone knows flax for its textile fibre. But the remarkable therapeutic and dietetic properties of its seed, rich both in fibre and polyunsaturated oil, are far less well known.

Linseed accelerates transit, lubricates stools and increases their size. It is an effective laxative, but gentle because a feature is that it also treats abdominal pains and colitis.

Finally, the oil contained in the seed (46%) is the one which contains the highest level of omega 3 essential fatty acids or EFAs, that are essential to life. Linseed oil helps to nourish the brain, fluidifies the membranes improving all the cell exchanges and nervous equilibrium, and reduces cholesterol levels. Also, because of omega 6 EFAs, it improves skin quality. For all these reasons, linseed is an excellent food, to be used daily, even in children.

Recommended for:
• High cholesterol.

DOSAGE
500mg per capsule of first cold pressed Organic Flax Oils

PHYTO PRESCRIPTION
Take 3 to 6 capsules daily with a large glass of water.
Contraindications/ Side-effects:
None known.

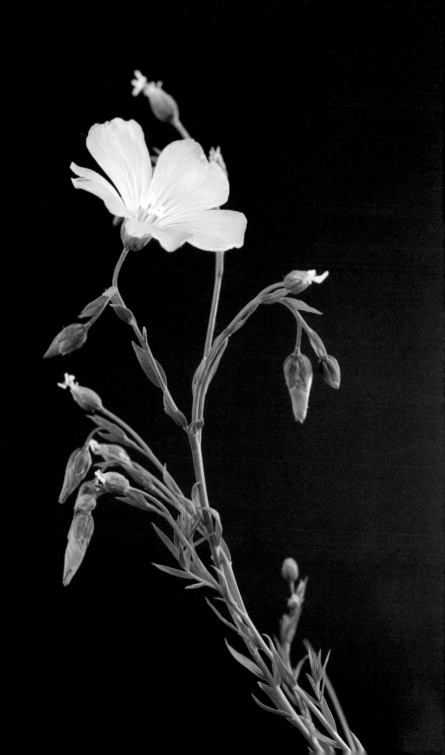

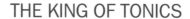

GINGER
Zingiber officinale

Part used: the rhizome

Ginger is one of the oldest Indian and Chinese remedies. Its rhizome has a characteristic and aromatic smell due to the essential oil and a spicy flavour. A few substances have been isolated, among them a particular group called gingerols, which give ginger its therapeutic properties. Studies that have been made on gingerols confirm its aphrodisiac reputation. They have also shown a beneficial action towards fertility, by increasing the amount of sperm produced and improving the sperms' mobility. Associated with Siberian ginseng, it reinforces its stimulating and energising activity. Ginger is also a good stomachic and is used for travel sickness. It helps improve digestion because it is a choleretic and a cholagogue, in other words it complements the secretion and the excretion of bile.

Recommended for:
- Sexual tiredness, impotence and asthenia
- Travel sickness
- Nausea
- Difficult digestion

DOSAGE
365mg per capsule of total plant cryoground powder

PHYTO PRESCRIPTION
Take 1 capsule 3 times a day during meals with a large glass of water. When travelling take 2 capsules half an hour before journey. Children (5-12 years): 1 capsule.

Contraindications/ Side-effects:
None known.

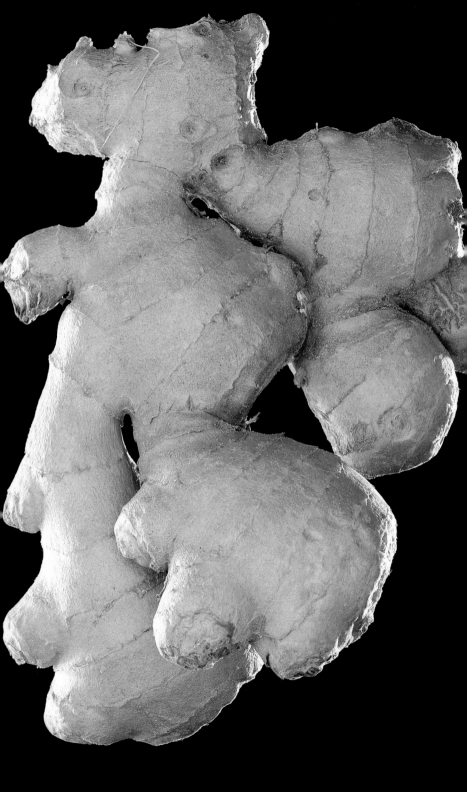

BENEFICIAL FOR THE MEMORY AND ALERTNESS

GINKGO
Ginkgo biloba

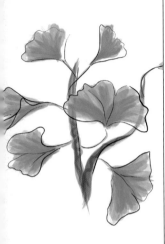

Part used: the leaf
250mg per capsule of total plant cryoground powder

Sacred tree of the Asian temples, Ginkgo is a true living fossil, which has stayed the same for over 250 million years. It has adapted itself to today's pollution and can live for thousand of years. Its fan-shaped leaves contain very active flavonoids. They have antioxidant activity and help capture the free radicals at the retinal and cerebral level.

Ginkgo helps decrease the ageing process of the retina and problems linked to senescence. Ginkgo regulates capillary permeability. It is a vasodilatator and helps reduce blood viscosity.

Numerous clinical trials have shown the efficacy of Ginkgo for improving blood circulation. It is an excellent treatment for cerebral ageing, it improves the memory, vigilance and moods. It is therefore beneficial for both peripheral and cerebral circulation. With its veinotonic action, it could be recommended to women who are taking the contraceptive pill to help reduce circulatory problems.

Recommended for:
• Fighting against the ageing process.
• Cerebral circulation problems: memory loss, tinnitus (ringing in the ears)
• Vertigo
• Peripheral circulation.

DOSAGE
250mg per capsule of total plant cryoground powder

PHYTO PRESCRIPTION
1 capsule morning, noon and evening with meals with a large glass of water.
Contraindications/ Side-effects:
None known.

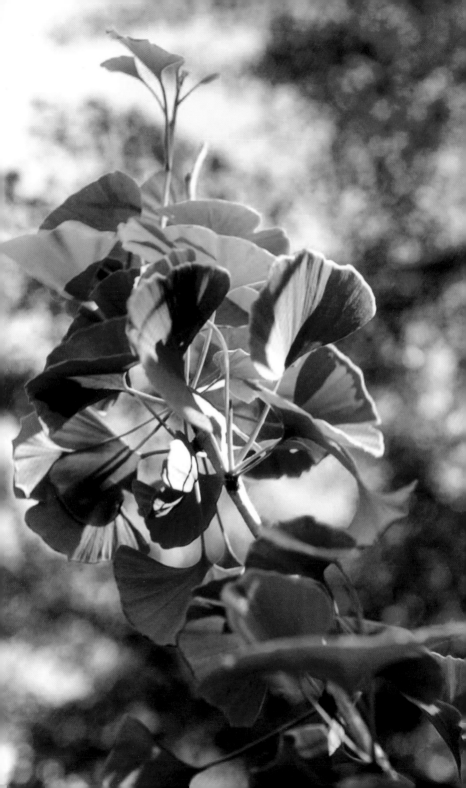

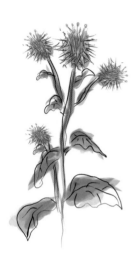

GREAT BURDOCK
Arctium lappa

Part used: the root

This robust and biennial plant from temperate areas grows in glades. This plant has a very long root which is rich in polyenes and alcohol acids, which explains its therapeutic activities.

Great Burdock has a skin depurative action and therefore a cleansing effect. Also the phenol-acids help to eliminate toxins in the liver and kidneys by means of their choleretic and diuretic action.

The polyenes act as anti-bacterial and antifungal agents, so reinforcing its depurative action.

Therefore, the root of the Great burdock is used for the treatment of acne, eczema, furunculosis (boils) and other dermatological disorders.

Recommended for:
- Acne
- Eczema
- Furunculosis (boils)
- Stimulation of the elimination functions of the liver and the kidneys
- Additional treatment for diabetes

DOSAGE
350mg per capsule of total plant cryoground powder

PHYTO PRESCRIPTION
Take 1 capsule morning, noon and evening before meals with a large glass of water. The intake can be increased to 5 capsules per day.

Contraindications/ Side-effects:
None known.

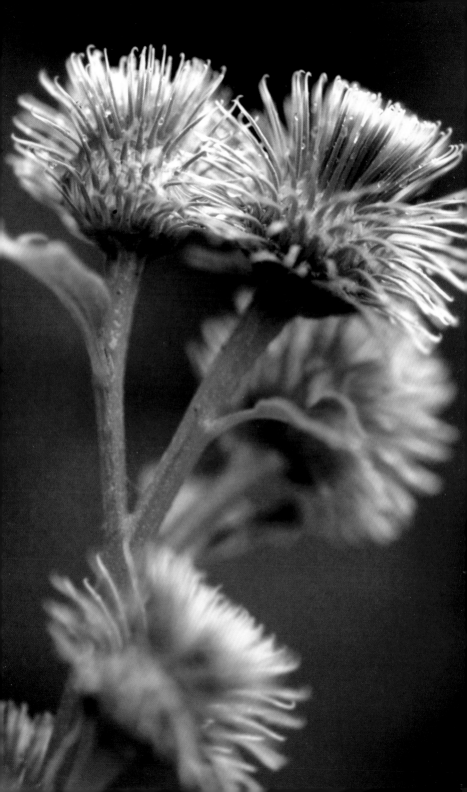

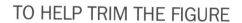

GREEN TEA
Camellia sinensis

Part used: the buds and the first 2 leaves of the branches

This tree originate s from India and was dis covered by the E uropeans in t he seventeenth century. Once its leaves have been fermented, a well-appreciated drink can be prepared, a drink which was originally called by the Indians the "Imperial Drink". In phytotherapy, the young leaves and buds of green tea can be used for slimming diets. Only the non- fermented leaves and buds are used to keep the integrity of the active ingredients. The leaves are of a beautiful da rk gree n and have a very int eres ting lipolysis activity. T he caff eine co ntent promotes draining of the fat outside the adipose tissues (fatty cells), by enzymatic stimulation: the triglycerides that are stored are then mobilised as free soluble fatty acids and therefore are easily eliminated by the body. The polyphenol content in green tea has a double interest: it permits a progressive liberation of the caffeine, therefore avoiding any ner vous and sleeping problems, and can also d ecrease the a ssimi lation of food carbohydrates and lipids and thus limits calorie intake.

Recommended for:
• Obesity and overweight
• Tiredness due to slimming

Remember: for dieting, it can only be used with a calorie controlled diet.

DOSAGE
390mg per capsule of total plant cryoground powder

PHYTO PRESCRIPTION
1 capsule morning, noon and evening with meals with a large glass of water.

Contraindications/ Side-effects:
None known.
Pregnant/breast feeding women should consult their doctor.

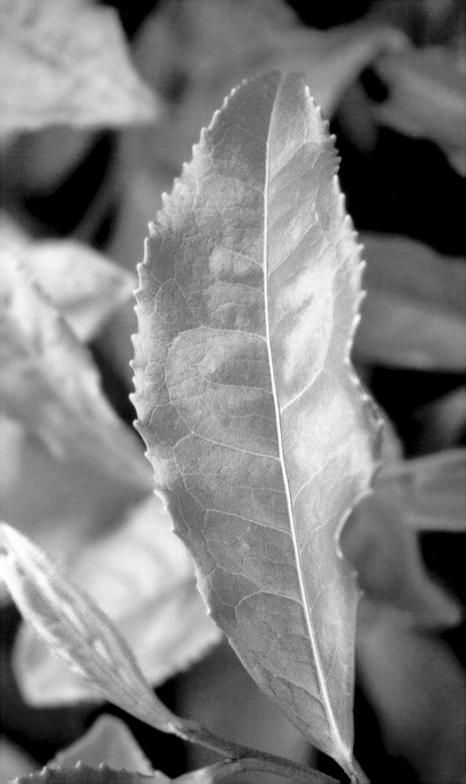

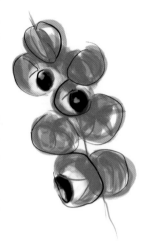

GUARANA
Paullinia cupana

Part used: the seed

This bush comes from the Amazon and is used a lot in Brazil by the Guarani Indians. The seeds are collected, roasted, crushed and mixed with water to make a stimulating drink.

Of all known plants, Guarana is the one which contains most caffeine. Caffeine helps increase the metabolism of cells and activate the combustion of fat. It also helps stimulate adrenaline which allows the body to burn fat faster. So, we can say that Guarana is particularly useful during dieting.

By increasing the release of adrenaline, it has a very stimultating effect on the body, helping to improve the body's resistance. Guarana can also be used for the treatment of physical or psychological asthenia, which often follows a slimming programme.

Recommended for:
- Obesity and overweight
- Physical and psychological asthenia
- Convalescence

Remember for weight loss, it can only be used with a calorie controlled diet.

DOSAGE
445mg per capsule of total plant cryoground powder

PHYTO PRESCRIPTION
Take 1 capsule morning, noon and evening during meals with a large glass of water.

Contraindications/ Side-effects:
None known.

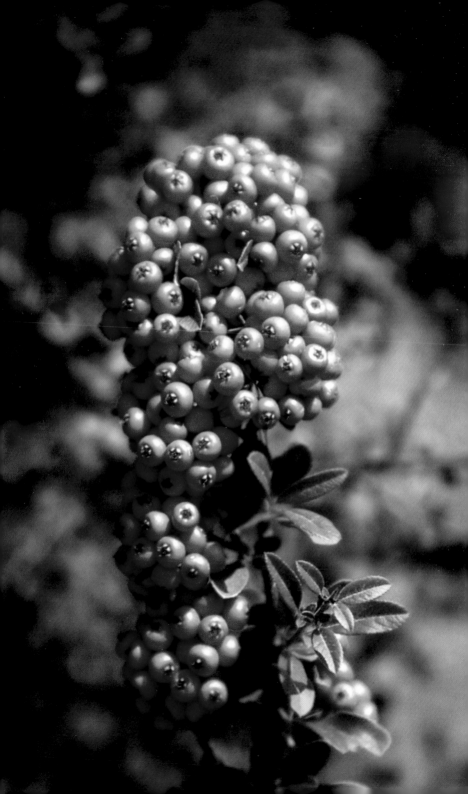

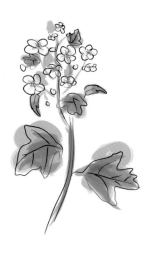

HAWTHORN
Crataegus Oxyacantha

Part used: aerial flowering part

Hawthorn fruit has long been used as a food and medication in Europe; particular is the name for bushes and small trees in the genus Crataegus, of which there are approximately 280 species native to northern temperate zones in East Asia, Europe and eastern North America. Over the past 20 years, several different commercially available preparations of hawthorn have been investigated in double-blind, placebo-controlled clinical studies. The flavonoids present, notably hyperoside and vitexin, regulate heart rate; consequently they act on excessively rapid rates, reduce heart palpitations and the exaggerated perception of heartbeats by people suffering from anxiety. It is a cardiac tonic, which supports tired hearts. Hawthorn has a dilatory effect on the coronary arteries and thus helps to prevent attacks of angina pectoris. It also reduces nervousness and anxiety in adults and children, treats sleep disorders and improves heart rate disorders in spasmophilics.

Recommended for:
- Reducing heart palpitations
- Anxiety and sleep problems
- Supporting tired hearts

DOSAGE
350mg of total cryoground powder of Hawthorn.

PHYTO PRESCRIPTION
Take 1 capsule morning, noon and evening during meals and with a large glass of water. The dose can be increased to a total of 5 capsules per day, if necessary.

Contraindications:
None known.

Pregnancy and Lactation:
No known restrictions, but no scientific data currently exists.

Drug interactions:
Consult your doctor before combining hawthorn with any heart medication.

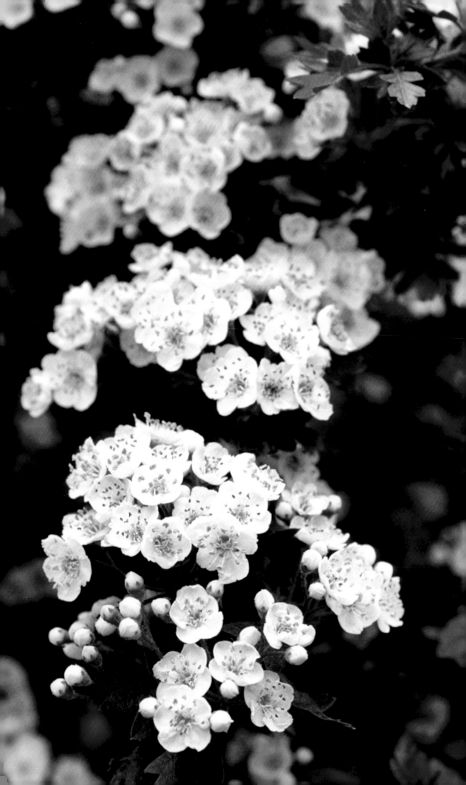

ISPAGHULA
Plantago ovata

Part used: the seed husks

Ispaghula is a plant belonging to the Plantaginacea family which often grows in Pakistan and India. The teguments of the seeds are rich in mucilage. This forms in the stomach, when mixed with cold water, a gel which is not assimilated by the organism but which has multiple benefits. Ispaghula is particularly appreciated during slimming diets for two main reasons: firstly, it naturally takes the edge off hunger; secondly it slows down the absorption of food during digestion, especially sugar and fat, thereby minimizing calorie intake. This high viscosity gel is beneficial to re-educate the intestinal tract which breaks the vicious circle of "classic" laxatives. It increases the volume and the hydration of the stools, making their elimination easier. Also, by covering the intestine walls, it has a protective action. This gel can also absorb bile salts which will then be evacuated along with the stools instead of being held within the intestine. So, the liver will have to use cholesterol to make more bile salts and in this way Ispaghula will reduce the cholesterol and triglyceride levels.

Recommended for:
• Slimming diets (helps reduce the appetite and slows down the absorption of food)
• Constipation
• Helps lower cholesterol and triglyceride levels (reducing their absorption)

Please remember for slimming: can only be used with a calorie controlled diet.

DOSAGE
430mg per capsule of total plant cryoground powder

PHYTO PRESCRIPTION
Take 2 capsules with a large glass of water before each meal. The intake can be increased to 4 capsules.

Contraindications/ Side-effects:
Not recommended in case of abdominal pains. Long term use should be approved by your practitioner.

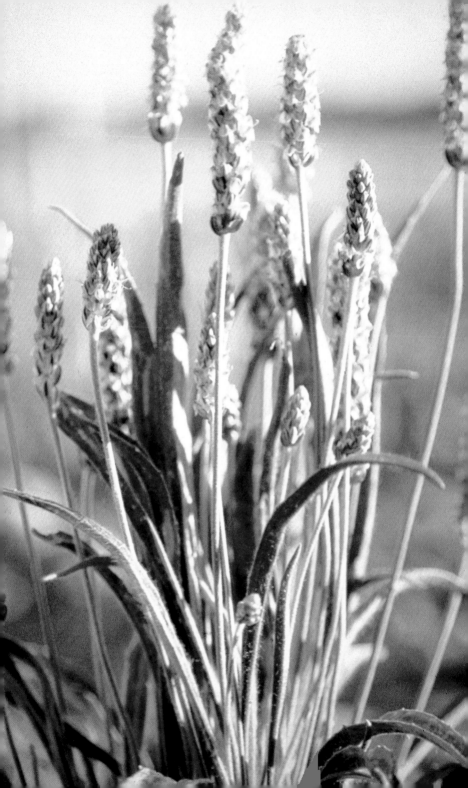

MILK THISTLE
Silybum marianum

Part used: fruit

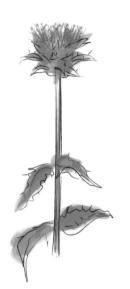

Milk thistle gets its name from a medieval legend. The Virgin Mary, wanting to conceal her baby Jesus from Herod's soldiers, hid him under the big leaves of a thistle. In her haste, a few drops of milk fell from her breast on to the thistle leaves, which have retained a hereditary trace of it close to their ribs. The basic plant for the liver: From a more scientific viewpoint, the fruit of this plant contains three substances (silybin, silychristin, silydanin) that are beneficial to the liver and are covered by the generic name silymarin. Silymarin is a liver protector: it contributes to a speedier recovery from hepatitis and cirrhosis by promoting liver reconstruction. It aids gall bladder flow and is thus active in cases of hepatic insufficiency or gallstones. Combined with fumitory, it provides an excellent liver drainage effect. Milk thistle is also haemostatic. It is therefore recommended for frequent

Recommended for:
- Hepatic insufficiency
- Gallstone
- Heavy periods

DOSAGE
300mg per capsule of total plant cryoground powder

PHYTO PRESCRIPTION
1 capsule morning, midday and evening, to be taken at mealtimes.
**Contraindications/
Side-effects:**
None known.

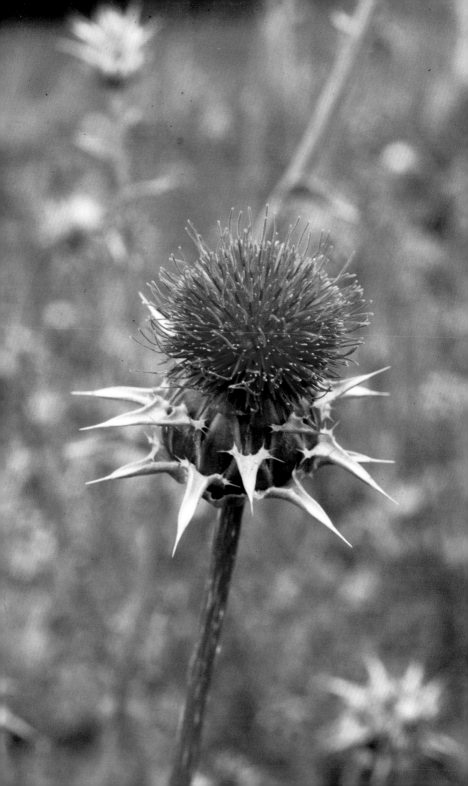

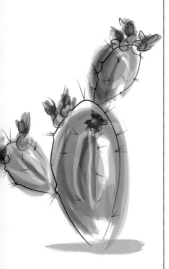

NOPAL CACTUS
Opuntia Ficus Indica

Part used: Stem

Nopal Cactus, also known as the Prickly Pear Cactus, is a member of the Cactus family. Nopal is currently cultivated in Mexico, Chile and Italy.

Nopal Cactus contains a high content of gums and mucilage, giving it the unique ability to bind to fats and sugars consumed during meals and reduce their digestion and absorption in the body. In addition to minimising the absorption of fats and sugars, Nopal Cactus also curbs the appetite and limits calorie intake by creating a feeling of satiety.

Nopal Cactus contains 17 amino acids, which provide you with additional energy, reduces fatigue by helping the body to lower blood sugar, improve mood, suppress appetite and provide nutrients. Nopal's vegetable protein helps the body transfer fluids from the tissues back into the bloodstream, thereby reducing cellulite and fluid retention.

Recommended for:
• Obesity and overweight.
• Tiredness that often occurs during calorie-controlled diets.

DOSAGE
500 mg per capsule of total plant cryoground powder

PHYTO PRESCRIPTION
Take one capsule during meals with a large glass of water. Take two capsules after heavy meals.

Contraindications/ Side-effects:
None known. Adults only. Pregnant/breast feeding women should consult their doctor.

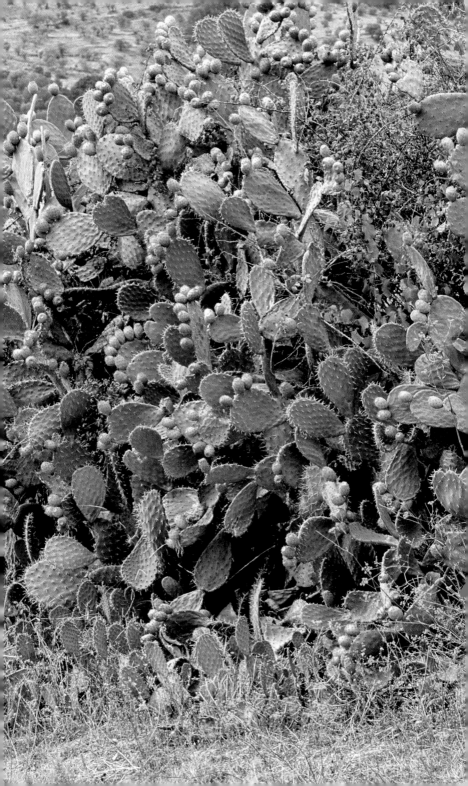

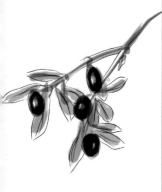

OLIVE
Olea europaea

Part used: leaf

Olive trees grow all around the Mediterranean, on dry, stony soils. The leaves are the active part because of the oleuropeoside that they contain. They are hypotensive and act on all the subjective disorders of hypertension: headaches, dizziness and ringing in the ears. Their direct action on hypertension is complemented by a diuretic effect. Olive tree is useful for the prevention of arteriosclerosis and coronary disease: it reduces bad cholesterol (LDL) levels and increases good cholesterol (HDL) levels. It also regulates heart rate. The leaf's safety (no contraindications or side-effects) and its proven efficacy make olive tree a preventive and curative treatment for hypertension. It has a hypoglycemic action and is therefore used as an adjuvant in the treatment of non-insulin-dependent diabetes.

Recommended for:
- Hypertension
- Cardiovascular diseases
- NID Diabetes

DOSAGE
275 mg per capsule of total plant cryoground powder

PHYTO PRESCRIPTION
1 capsule morning, midday and evening, to be taken at mealtimes.

**Contraindications/
Side-effects:**
None known.

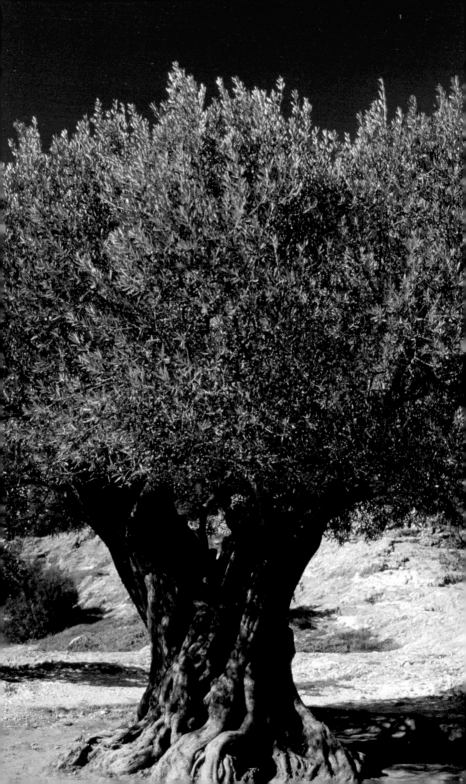

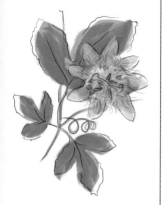

PASSIFLORA
Passiflora incarnata

Part used: the aerial part

Passiflora is a beautiful plant originally from Mexico, where it was used by the Aztecs for its sedative properties. It was brought into Europe by the Spanish Jesuits under the name of "Passion flower". They saw in the shape of the flower Christ's instrument of passion. The aerial part of the plant contains flavonoids which contribute to its beneficial action for sleeping problems. It progressively brings back natural sleep for insomniacs. It is very beneficial for anxiety and nervousness accumulated by a life full of stress and therefore prepares for a peaceful and restful sleep. It is neither addictive nor habit forming and can be used to replace progressively and substitute pharmaceutical classical remedies which we know can have long term side-effects.

Recommended for:
- Insomnia
- Agitation and anxiety
- Nervousness and stress
- Breaking the habit created by classical hypnotics and anxiolytics

DOSAGE
230 mg per capsule of total plant cryoground powder

PHYTO PRESCRIPTION
1 to 2 capsules during the day for the relief of the stresses and strains of modern living. 2 to 3 capsules after the evening meal to help promote natural sleep.

Contraindications/ Side-effects:
Not recommended during pregnancy.

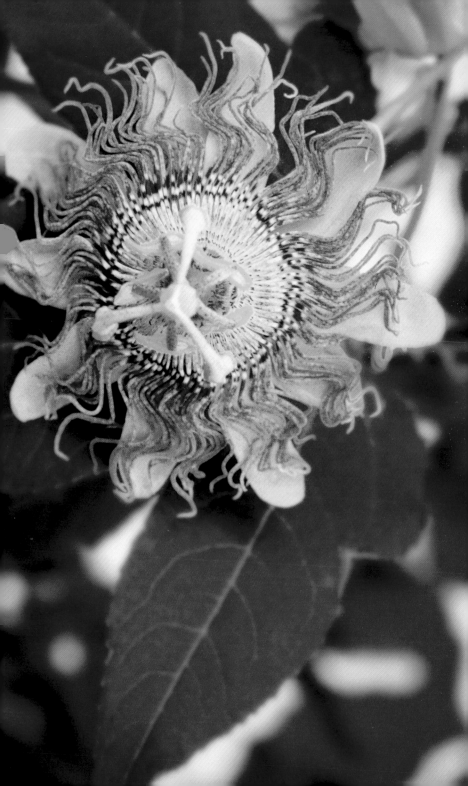

PINEAPPLE
Ananas comosus

Part used: the stem

This exotic fruit plant was discovered in Guadeloupe by Christopher Colombus in 1493. The natives called it "nana". It has been eaten for its taste for a long time. It contains a proteolytic enzyme called Bromelin which is essentially concentrated in the stem. This means that even an excessive consumption of the fruit won't give a total benefit of the Bromelin. So, the absorption of the whole plant powder of the stem in capsule form is very interesting. In fact, bromelin has an antiinflammatory action for the gradual reduction of localized oedema. Also this enzyme helps stop the rise of the insulin level in the blood (this level is increased when we eat sugar - i.e. cakes or ice-cream) and therefore the rise of fat reserves coming from sugar. The absorbed bromelin is released into the body, allowing a breakdown of the proteins not normally secreted at the tissue level (cellulite, bruising) into easily eliminated amino acids. This way, the appearance of the "dimpled orange skin" will decrease.

Recommended for:
- Cellulite
- Localised fat
- Oedema, bruising

Please remember for slimming, it can only be used with a calorie controlled diet.

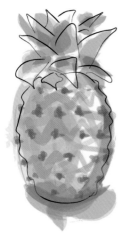

DOSAGE
400 mg per capsule of total plant cryoground powder

PHYTO PRESCRIPTION
Take 1 capsule morning, noon and evening after meals with a large glass of water.

Contraindications/ Side-effects:
None known.

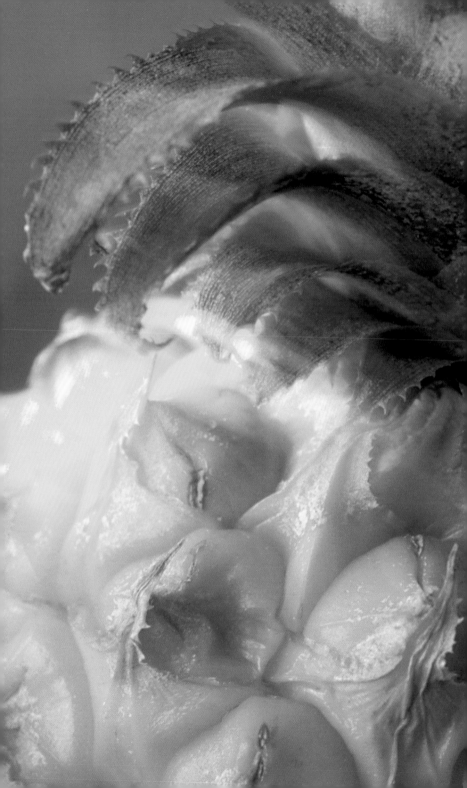

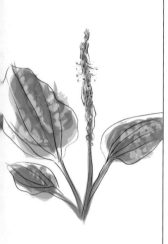

THE "ANTI-ALLERGY" PLANT FOR THE RESPIRATORY TRACT

COMMON PLANTAIN
Plantago major

Part used: the leaf

Common Plantain grows all over France, in the fields and footpaths. Its leaves are very tender when young and they form pretty rosettes on the ground. One of the principle iridoids found in its leaves is aucuboside, which has anti-bacterial and anti-tussive properties used to heal bronchial illnesses. Plantain leaves also contain mucilage which provides a softer and emollient action, and facilitates expectoration. Plantain is also used as an antiinflammatory and an anti-allergic. So, it is a very valuable addition for respiratory allergies.

Recommended for:
• Respiratory problems, due to allergies such as asthma, coughs, rhinitis, hay fever and sinusitis.
• Anti-inflammatory: bronchitis, pharyngitis and laryngitis.e

DOSAGE
280 mg per capsule of total plant cryoground powder

PHYTO PRESCRIPTION
Take 1 capsule morning, noon and evening during meals with a large glass of water.

Contraindications/ Side-effects:
None known.

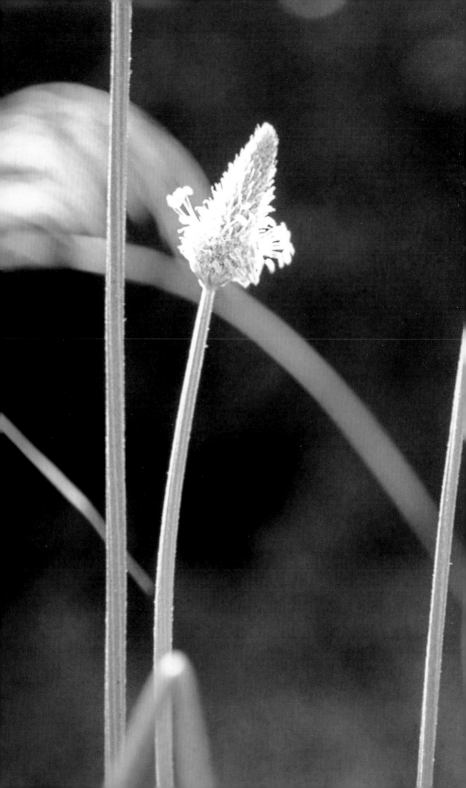

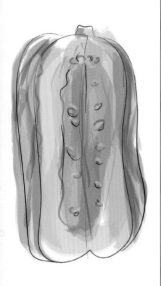

PUMPKIN SEED/ SAW PALMETTO

Paullinia cupana

Part used: The seed / Berries

Pumpkin seeds are a rich source of phytosterols. Phytosterols are natural steroids, which counteract hormonal changes that take place in the body of middle-aged men. Saw Palmetto is part of the Palm family and originates from the USA. Its berries were a popular food among Native Americans and settlers, who valued them for their tonic effect. Recent research has shown that Saw Palmetto not only helps to prevent benign prostate enlargement, but it also helps to cure the disorder. Because both Pumpkin seeds and Saw Palmetto inhibit the conversion of testosterone into dihydrotestosterone, which is believed to be responsible for enlargement of the prostate, this complex is highly valued by men. Indeed one in three men suffers from this disorder from the age of fifty on and one in two from the age of sixty. Pumpkin seed oil and Saw Palmetto are often associated with Zinc because Zinc is good not only for the immune system but also for the prostate gland.

Recommended for:
• Urinary and prostate disorders
• To stimulate the immune system

DOSAGE
Per 2 capsules: 80mg Pumpkin seed oil, 320mg Saw Palmetto berry oil extract, 15mg Zinc

PHYTO PRESCRIPTION
Take 1 capsule with both breakfast and lunch, to be swallowed with a large glass of water.

Contraindications/ Side-effects:
Medical advice should be sought if the condition persists or is accompanied by bleeding or a fever.

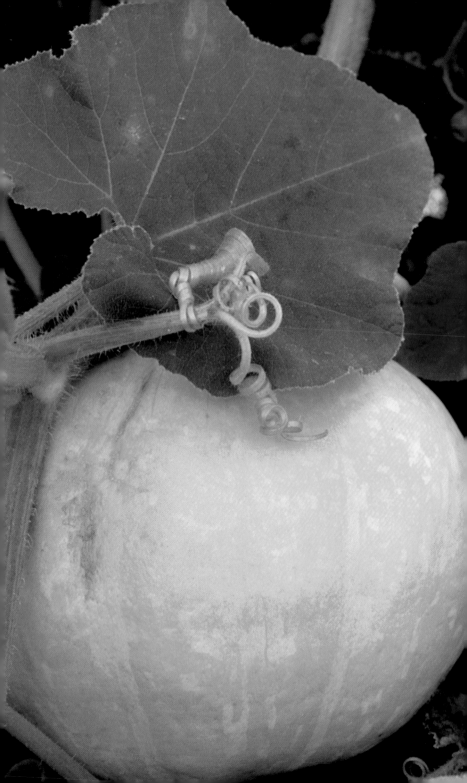

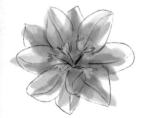

RHODIOLA
Rhodiola rosea

Part used: Root

There are at least 200 species of Rhodiola in the world and they differ in their chemical make-up.

The species Rhodiola rosea, is only found in a few remote areas in the northern regions of Europe, Scandinavia, Lapland and Alaska. Rhodiola, also known as rose root, golden root, and arctic root possesses properties that enable individuals to cope with everyday situations.

It is traditionally believed to give strength and stamina, as it is known to oxygenate the brain as well as muscle tissue, providing a dramatic boost in energy levels. It has been commonly used to treat long-term illness and tiredness due to infection, mood elevation, mental alertness, sports performance and weight loss.

Recommended for:
• Weight reduction
• Depression
• Maintaining energy levels
• Increasing attention span, memory and mental performance
• Increasing strength & mobility

DOSAGE
400mg of powdered Rhodiola root

PHYTO PRESCRIPTION
Take 2 capsules in the morning and 1 at midday during meals with a large glass of water.

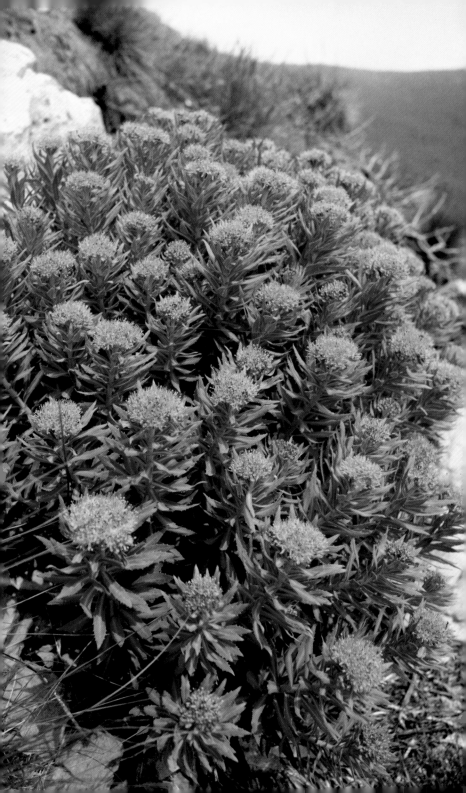

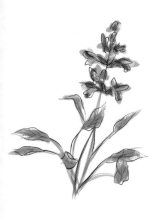

THE PLANT FOR DIFFICULT DIGESTION

SAGE
Salvia lavandulifolia

Part used: the leaf

It is said that those who have sage in their gardens have no need for a doctor. Sage (from the latin salvare which means "to save") has, since antiquity, been considered the universal panacea and was wellrecognized by the Greeks. The school of Salerne taught the many virtues of this plant. The leaves are rich in flavonoids and essential oil which explains its spicy taste and aromatic smell. Sage helps increase the secretion of bile and therefore acts as a choleretic. It has a relaxing and antispasmodic effect on the stomach and intestine muscles. The essential oil also acts as an antiseptic. These properties are particularly useful for digestive problems such as slow and difficult digestion, flatulence, intestinal fermentation and gas. Sage contains "plant" oestrogens and can so be recommended to women who suffer from irregular and painful periods and also during the menopause to reduce hot flushes. The essential oil acts on the sudoriferous glands which help reduce sweat formation which can be excessive during the menopause.

Recommended for:
- Difficult digestion
- Menstruation problems
- Menopausal hot flushes
- Excessive perspiration

DOSAGE
285mg per capsule of total plant cryoground powder

PHYTO PRESCRIPTION
Take 2 capsules morning and evening during meals with a large glass of water.
Contraindications/ Side-effects:
None known.

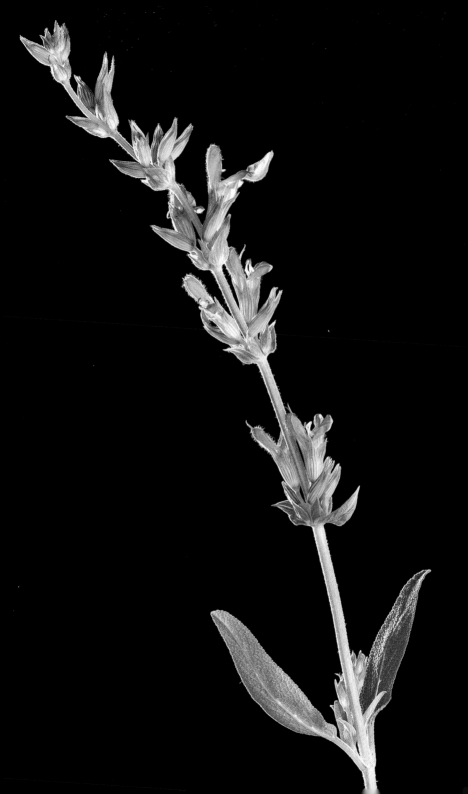

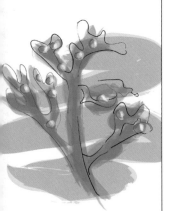

SEAWEED
Fucus vesiculosus

Part used: the thallus

Seaweed, which is a symbol of life, is a natural concentrate of the ocean richness. Collected manually at low tide, it is a real cocktail of vital elements. Seaweed actually provides all the trace elements contained in sea water; among them copper, chromium, zinc, selenium, iron, manganese, iodine (starter of the body reactions) and even gold in an infinitesimal quantity. It is a rich source of vitamins, such as folic acid, vitamin C, group B vitamins (thiamine, riboflavin, B6, B12) thus helping to metabolise nutrients, especially sugars. Seaweed is therefore of great nutritional interest and it stimulates cellular exchanges and the elimination of waste materials from the body.

Seaweed is rich in assimilated vegetable proteins and low in calories and fats. Furthermore, it contains non assimilated mucilage which swells in contact with water and distends the stomach, thus helping to reduce the appetite. The vegetable fibres have a laxatif effect. Seaweed is therefore recommended during a low calorie diet in order to reduce appetite and help the body lose weight while providing the body with all the essential elements necessary for its vitality and balance..

Recommended for:
- The suppression of hunger/reduction of appetite
- Low calorie diet
- Fatigue
- Helps weight loss

DOSAGE
130mg per capsule of total plant cryoground powder

PHYTO PRESCRIPTION
Adults: 1 capsule, 1 to 3 times daily for 3 weeks to be taken with a glass of water before meals. Not recommended for children below 12 years of age.

Contraindications/ Side-effects:

Not recommended for people with thyroid conditions. Not recommended during pregnancy.

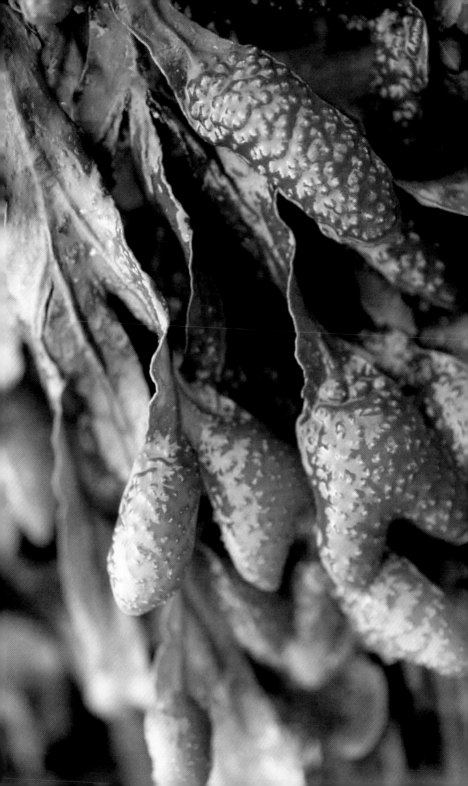

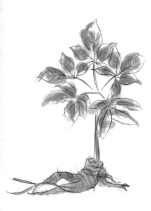

THE MOST VITAL INGREDIENT FOR ENERGY

SIBERIAN GINSENG
Eleutherococcus senticosus

Part used: the root

This plant is very common in Siberia and can also be found in certain areas of China and Korea. It is often called "Russia's secret plant" and is extensively used by sportsmen in Russia. Its root contains eleutherosides from which it gets its properties. Siberian Ginseng is an "adaptogen", which means that it acts on the body, favouring a harmonious adaptation to different situations. For example, Siberian Ginseng is used by Russian cosmonauts, helping their bodies adapt to space travel. Siberian Ginseng's roots also facilitate physical efforts, increasing the resistance capacity and improving the body's powers to recuperate. It has been used for many years by Russian athletes, and we are all aware of their magnificent performances in the Olympic games. This root is highly energizing and is a good tonic for males. The stimulating and energizing effect would be more easily explained by the hormonal control of the hypothalamus and the pituitary gland. Siberian Ginseng also facilitates intellectual concentration. The organism's increased resistance will be constantly maintained, even after the treatment. Siberian Ginseng is a chosen ally to homoeopathic treatments as it stimulates the defence reactions without substituting them.

Recommended for:
- Physical or intellectual fatigue (overwork)
- Preparation for sporting activities
- Tonic for males
- Preparation for school exams
- Convalescence

DOSAGE
250mg per capsule of total plant cryoground powder

PHYTO PRESCRIPTION
Take 2 capsules mornings and noon during meals with a large glass of water. Intake can be increased to 6 capsules per day.
Contraindications/ Side-effects:
None known.

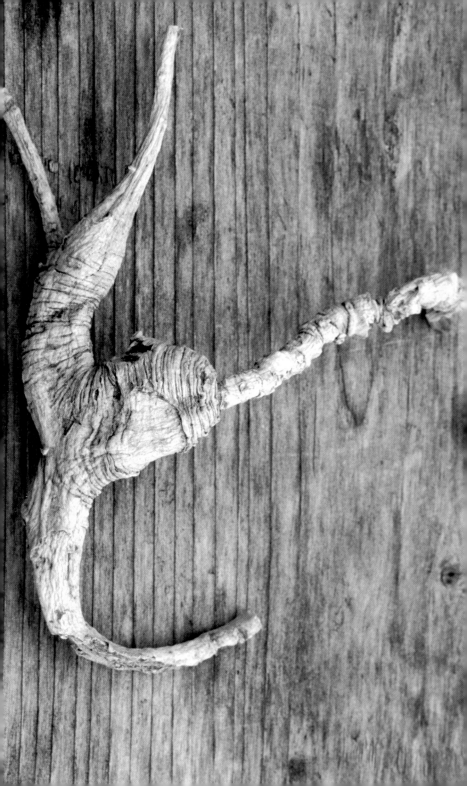

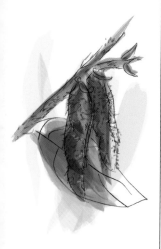

FOR THE IMPROVED URINARY COMFORT OF MEN OVER THE AGE OF 50

SOYA ISOFLAVONES
Semen sojae - Plant sterols - Zinc

Part used: Soya beans Concentrate of plant oils rich in sterols Zinc

Numerous studies demonstrate that Soya Isoflavones can assist in normal prostate health, urinary flow, and quality of life of men, particularly those over 50. In Japan where a lot of soy is consumed, typically 20-40mg of Isoflavones derived from soybeans daily, prostate problems are more rare than in 'western men', where very little amounts are consumed Sterols are one of the most studied natural ingredients for their positive influence on urinary function. Zinc is known to be an integral part of the structure of male hormones and is a major constituent of seminal fluid. Soya Isoflavones, Plant Sterol Extract and Zinc represent an excellent combination to prevent and treat urinary problems resulting from the common prostate problem BPH (Benign Prostatic Hyperplasia or Benign Prostate Hypertrophy), a noncancerous enlargement of the prostate that restricts the flow of urine from the bladder. BPH is a common problem that affects millions of men over the age of 50. Soya Isoflavones, Plant Sterols and Zinc are an excellent combination for those patients with mild and moderate symptoms, surgery being chosen by patients suffering from severe symptoms.

Recommended for:
- Urinary problems resulting from Benign Prostate
- Hyperplasia (BPH)

PHYTO PRESCRIPTION
1 capsule morning and evening during meals with a large glass of water.
Contraindications/ Side-effects:
None known.

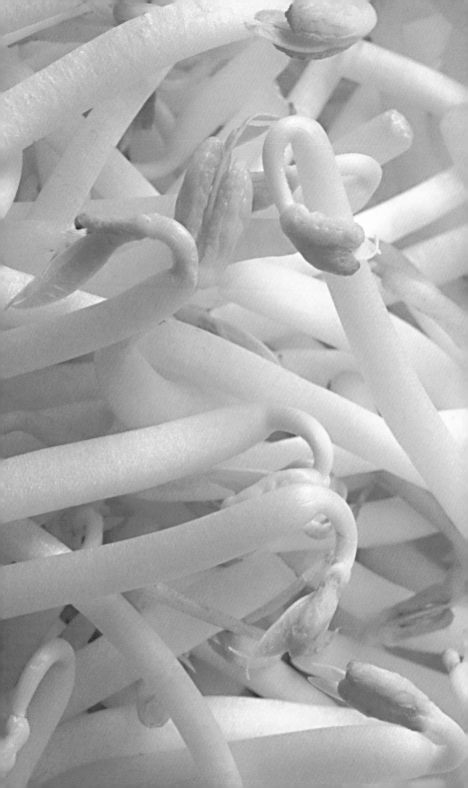

SOYA SAPONINS

Part used: soya beans

Soya Saponins are a dietetic food supplement intended for those wishing to help prevent harmful effects of sodium. Saponins are abundant in Soya beans and also in green bean, broad beans, lentils and chick peas.

Soya contains more than eight varieties of saponins. It is accepted that they are an effective class of substances that activate the potassium channels. In the body each cell contains a sodium-potassium pump. This Na-K pump is indispensable for the good functioning of our cells, as it assists in regulating the sodium-potassium balance.

When the Na-K pump slows down there is an accumulation of sodium. A blocked cell can lead to malfunction of organs possibly leading to symptoms associated with high blood pressure, fatigue and irritable bowel syndrome.

Recommended for:
- Hypertension
- Type 2 diabetes
- Obesity
- Depression
- Fatigue and lack of energy
- Fluid retention

DOSAGE
250mg of extract rich in saponins

PHYTO PRESCRIPTION
Take 1 capsule morning and evening with a large glass of water. The dose can be increased to 4 capsules per day.

Contraindications/ Side-effects:
None known.

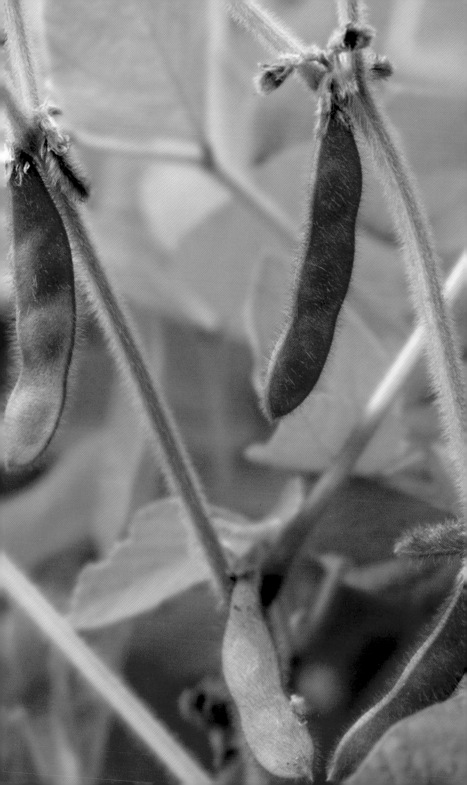

A PLANT FOR THE SKIN

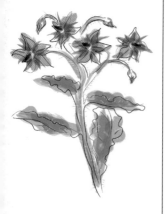

STARFLOWER OIL
Borago officinalis

Part used: the oil extracted from the seeds

Originating from the Middle East, this plant is also widespread in Central Europe and the Mediterranean countries. In the past its pretty blue flowers were used as an herbal tea when suffering from sore throat as they have excellent soothing powers.

Nowadays, the oil extracted from the seeds by cold pressing is extremely valuable due to its rich source of two polyunsaturated Essential Fatty Acids; Gamma Linolenic Acid and Linoleic Acid. Taken in capsule form, Starflower oil helps to fight against the ageing process of the skin and prevent the formation of wrinkles.

It improves the elasticity of the skin and makes it more resistant to outside aggressions. It also improves brittle nails and hair. To take full advantage of its benefits, Starflower oil should be taken regularly.

Recommended for:
- Wrinkles, dry skin, stretch marks
- Prevention of ageing process of the skin

DOSAGE

520mg per capsule of first cold pressed Starflower oil

PHYTO PRESCRIPTION

Internal usage: take 1 capsule a day, with a large glass of water. External usage: The capsule can be pierced and the oil applied to the skin.

Contraindications/ Side-effects:

None known.

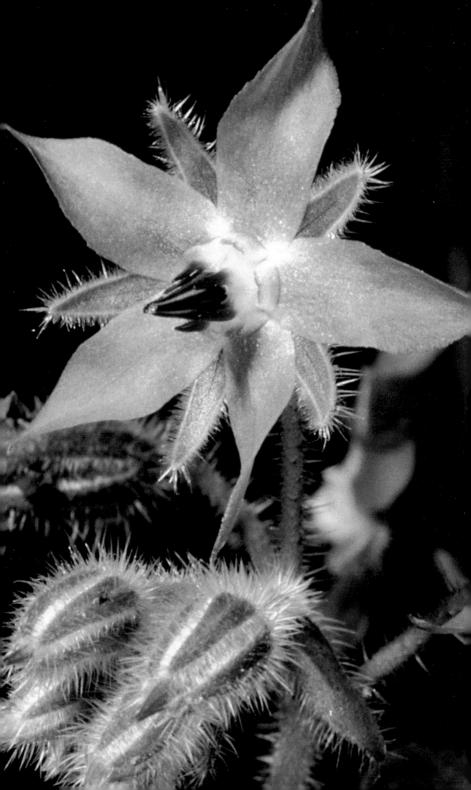

STINGING NETTLE
Urtica dioica

Part used: the aerial part

It is said that those who have sage in their gardens have no need for a doctor. Sage (from the latin salvare which means "to save") has, since antiquity, been considered the universal panacea and was wellrecognized by the Greeks. The school of Salerne taught the many virtues of this plant. The leaves are rich in flavonoids and essential oil which explains its spicy taste and aromatic smell. Sage helps increase the secretion of bile and therefore acts as a choleretic. It has a relaxing and antispasmodic effect on the stomach and intestine muscles. The essential oil also acts as an antiseptic. These properties are particularly useful for digestive problems such as slow and difficult digestion, flatulence, intestinal fermentation and gas. Sage contains "plant" oestrogens and can so be recommended to women who suffer from irregular and painful periods and also during the menopause to reduce hot flushes. The essential oil acts on the sudoriferous glands which help reduce sweat formation which can be excessive during the menopause.

Recommended for:
- Brittle nails and hair loss (a six-month course)
- Acne
- Fatigue and convalescence.

DOSAGE
275 mg per capsule of total plant cryoground powder

PHYTO PRESCRIPTION
Take 2 capsules morning and evening before meals with a large glass of water.
Contraindications/ Side-effects:
None known.

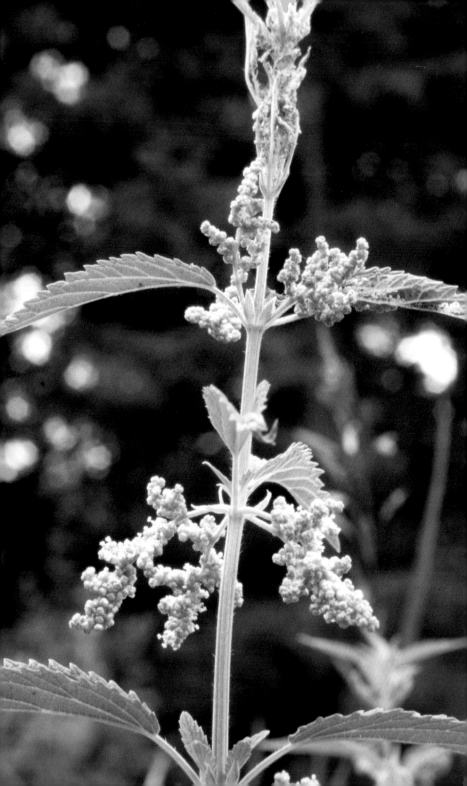

A PLANT FOR THE MIND

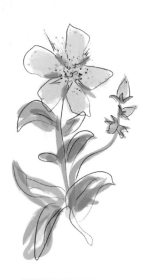

ST JOHN'S WORT
Hypericum perforatum

Part used: the flowering tip

St John's wort is an herbaceous plant often found on the footpaths of Europe, America and Northern Africa. Its leaves have a multiplicity of tiny secretory pockets which give the impression that they have been perforated.

The part used is the flowering tips, which are picked at the beginning of the summer around the St John's celebration, hence its name. St John's wort has been used for centuries and we can trace its use back to the 6th century when it was then used topically for the treatment of wounds and burns.

It was used in this manner for hundreds of years until the end of the last century when an American scientist described the plant as beneficial for the treatment of mild depression. Recently, clinical studies have highlighted the fact that St John's wort has a stimulant effect on the nervous system, due mainly to its active ingredient, xantone.

This makes St John's wort a very interesting plant when treating occasional depression.

Recommended for:
• Depression

DOSAGE
185mg standardised extract per capsule corresponding to 500µg hypericin

PHYTO PRESCRIPTION
Take 1 capsule at breakfast and 1 at lunch time with a large glass of water.

Contraindications/ Side-effects:
Those currently on antidepressant medication should ideally seek medical advice before using this herb. Prolonged exposure to the sun whilst on Hypericum should be avoided. Consult your doctor if you are on the contraceptive pill.

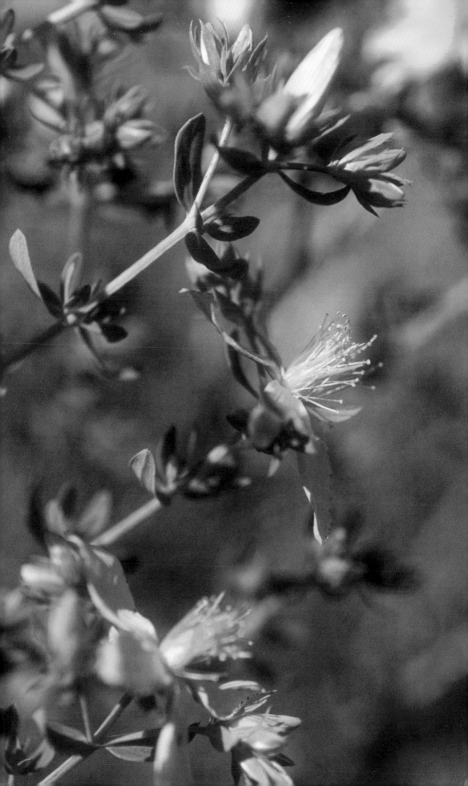

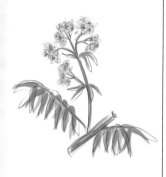

VALERIAN
Valeriana officinalis

Part used: the roots

At the beginning of the summer in the south of Europe, Valerian bushes of pink-purple colour flowers, can be seen on embankments and old walls. When the Valerian plant has been dried, it has a very particular odour which attracts cats !

The root (from latin valere which means "to be well") contains an essential oil and valepotriates (valtrate and isovaltrate) which both have a very effective and gentle sedative action. Valerian is used with great success for insomnia, anxiety and anguish, but without causing any addiction or drowsiness during the day.

When combined with the classical epilepsy treatment it helps the everyday life of epileptic people by contributing to the prevention of attacks (Valerian is recognized as an anti-convulsant and anti-epileptic).

It can also be used to help smokers give up the habit as it prevents feelings of nervousness and gives to bacco an unpleasant taste.

Recommended for:
- Insomnia
- Anti smoking
- Anxiety and anguish
- Can complement the treatment of epileptics

DOSAGE

270mg per capsule of total plant cryoground powder

PHYTO PRESCRIPTION

Adults: *Insomnia*: Take 2 capsules evenings before meals and 2 capsules before going to bed. *Nervousness*: Take 1 capsule morning, noon and evenings during meals. **Children:** Take 1 capsule evenings and 1 capsule before going to bed if sleep problems exist.

Contraindications/ Side-effects:

Not recommended for patients with liver impairment or on other medication known to have potential for liver toxicity or induction of liver enzymes. Not recommended during pregnancy.

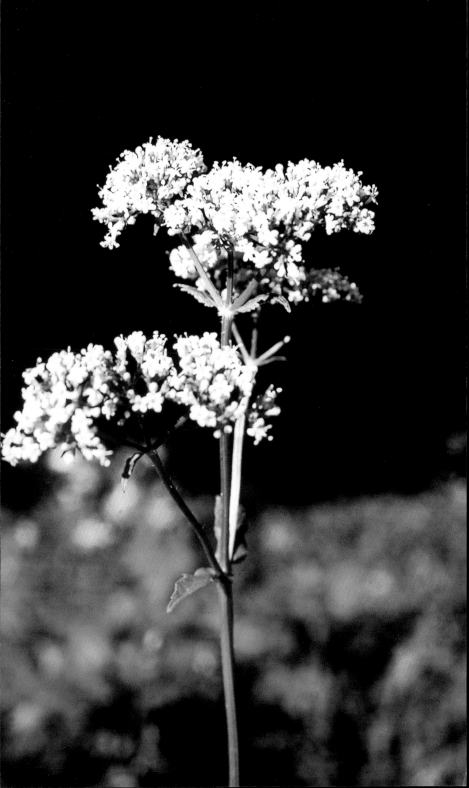

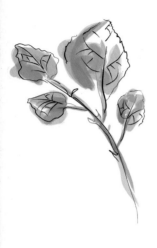

THE PLANT FOR THE FRAGILITY OF CAPILLARY TISSUES

WITCH HAZEL
Hamamelis virginiana

Part used: the leaf

This shrub comes from North America and its leaves are widely used for all circulatory disorders. Its composition is very interesting because it is rich in flavonoids and condensed tannins called proanthocyanidins.

This gives Witch hazel a double action on circulation: a tonic action on the veins due to its tannins and the properties of vitamin P due to its flavonoids. Vitamin P increases the resistance of capillary tissues and regulates their permeability, having at the same time an anti-inflammatory effect. Witch hazel is recommended for reduction of venous oedema, and with its tonic action it will be of benefit in the treatment of varicose veins, tired and heavy legs and will help relieve haemorrhoids.

The activity of vitamin P coupled with the protective action of proanthocyanidins is very useful for the improvement of the capillary vessels which can burst under the skin. Flavonoids are major antioxidants that protect the blood vessel walls.

Recommended for:
- Skin blotches
- Fragility of the small blood vessels
- Heavy legs
- Haemorrhoids
- Varicose veins

DOSAGE
290mg per capsule of total plant cryoground powder

PHYTO PRESCRIPTION
Take 1 capsule morning, noon and evening during meals with a large glass of water. Intake can be increased to 6 capsules per day.v

Contraindications/ Side-effects:
None known.

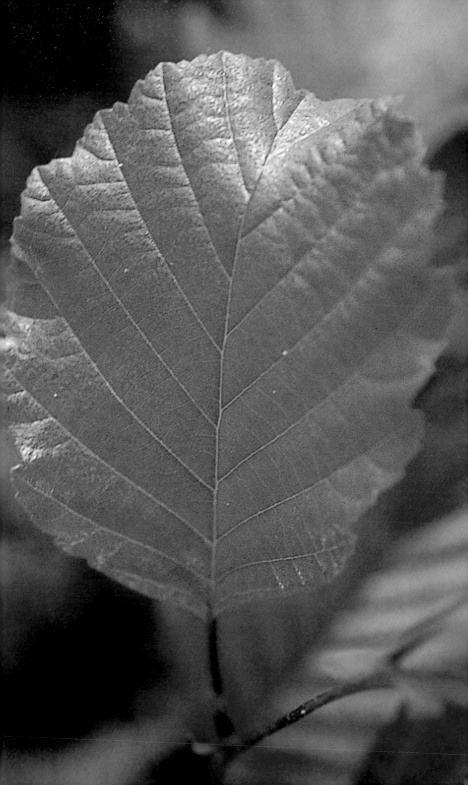

Also available at Alpen éditions

The Diet & Cookbooks Series:
Montignac Diet Cookbook
Montignac French Diet for Weight Loss
Eat Yourself Slim
Food Healing
Forever Young
The Anti Cholesterol Diet
The French GI Diet for Women
Osteoarthritis, Rheumatism, Arthritis

The Health books Series:
All About the Prostate
Control your Acidity: The Acid-Base Diet
Handle your Menopause
Herbal Healing
Living with a Hyperactive Child
Montignac Glycemix Index Diet
Omega-3 Answer
Osteoporosis
The French Paradox
The Paleo Diet
The XXL Syndrome

www.alpen.mc